Letters from the Land of Cancer

Books by Walter Wangerin Jr.

Letters from the Land of Cancer

Walter Wangerin Jr.

National Book Award Winning Author

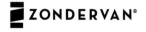

ZONDERVAN.com/
AUTHORTRACKER
follow your favorite authors

ZONDERVAN

Library of Congress Cataloging-in-Publication Data

Wangerin, Walter.
    Letters from the land of cancer / Walter Wangerin, Jr.
      p.   cm.
    ISBN 978-0-310-29281-4 (hardcover, jacketed)
    1. Wangerin, Walter. 2. Terminally ill—Religious life. 3. Lungs—Cancer—Patients—
Religious life. 4. Lungs—Cancer—Religious aspects—Christianity. I. Title.
BV4910.33.W36 2010
242'.4—dc22   2009040179

Cover design: Curt Diepenhorst

Interior design: Christine Orejuela-Winkelman

Printed in the United States of America

09 10 11 12 13 14 15 • 22 21 20 19 18 17 16 15 14 13 12 11 10 9 8 7 6 5 4 3 2 1

For my sister-in-law, Dorothy Bohlmann,
who made her dying
a radiant witness

Contents

Part Two

Prologue

This Kind of Cancer Doesn't Go Away

Now, AS I SIT TO write these words, I have cancer.

I call myself the "Professional Patient" for the amounts of time I spend with doctors, lying under their searching examinations, sitting before their estimations, their opinions and their consultations. *Professional* Patient, I say, for the even vaster amounts of time I must spend in their waiting rooms, waiting for examinations and consultations.

Cancer kicks off a swarm of symptoms and conditions which vary from patient to patient. Not all of one's secondary troubles could be predicted or even clearly explained once they've arrived. It's the body whole that takes the shock. Hence the large array of specialized physicians necessary for treatment. Besides the chemical oncologists and the radiologists and the family doctor, I have had to keep regular appointments with a pulmonologist, an ear, nose and throat specialist, a dentist, a psychologist; returning weekly and biweekly to the hospital and to various laboratories for blood tests, CT scans, PET scans, simple X-rays, physical therapies; constant traffic to the pharmacist, constantly rattling pills morning and evening—and "I'm prescribing oxygen. Here's where you can get it."

I have cancer. It's a business. It initiates one into its own peculiar community. It encounters a host of attitudes and personalities among its medical practitioners.

One of the bluntest said to me, "Have they prepared you?"

"Who? For what?"

"Have your attending physicians been direct with you regarding your cancer?"

"Well, I think so." I rattled off the cool, stainless-steel-like, scientific diagnoses which I had received already from my "attending physicians."

The doctor who was speaking to me at that particular moment is a short, grim, aggressive sort, lunging headfirst when he walks, tick-ticking away at his laptop even while he's talking to a patient. He commands that piece of equipment as much by the hard glare in his eye as by his flying fingers. It was the same glare that met me then.

"That's not what I mean. Have they prepared *you*? Your *heart* for what must come of the cancer you have?"

I blinked.

Without hesitation, without modulating his voice, lunge-talking onward, the doctor said:

"This kind of cancer doesn't go away. It will kill you. Sooner or later, this will be the cause of your death——"

——so long as other causes don't beg to be first.

I have cancer. It has dominated the time of my outward living. It has put death central inside of me. It isn't going away. For this there is no "cure."

On the other hand, my tumors——though present——have slowed their metabolic activities so much that I and my physicians have entered a waiting game, a period of watching whether the cancer shall have jumped back to a busier life again.

It is in this time of surcease that I find it both good and possible to look back over the past two years of my experience with cancer and, thereby, with my approaching death. Perhaps my story will give shape and meaning to the stories of so many people who are involved with terminal conditions: those sick, those who love and comfort the sick——and even those who for other reasons find themselves thinking deeply of death, and of their own deaths particularly.

Here is the story which must ultimately embrace every living body, every physical person. Here, too, is the story in which our faith in Christ most can shine. Such faith will surprise the most faithful. A patient thinks she will be afraid to die——but then she finds herself (astonishingly!) peaceful at the prospect, simply because there has never before been such an opportunity to test, to prove, to discover the real quality, of her faith, which is the presence of the Holy Spirit in her.

Let my story become your story too.

I'LL TELL MY STORY STEP-BY-STEP *from within* the ongoing experience. I needn't draw upon memory.

Shortly after the cancer had been diagnosed I began writing letters to the members of my immediate family, to relatives and to lifelong friends. I wrote with news almost immediately after I myself had heard the news. I wrote even while sitting in the oncologist's easy chair, receiving an infusion of the chemicals which would eventually take my hair and leave a scalp as bright and white as the moon.

The following book will consist mostly of those letters. They will invite you into my most intimate dance with the cancer, even as that partner and I have over the last two years swung each other around the tiled floors of ballrooms and bathrooms. Dizzy still, and day by day, I sat and wrote: *This is what I'm feeling right now. This is what I think.*

Hence the title: *Letters from the Land of Cancer.* The letters will be given you in the same sequence in which they were written.

With your indulgence, my friend, I will offer among these letters a number of more immediate observations, some reminiscences from my earlier life, and a few briefer, more pointed tales on the subject of this final, most common experience of every soul born flesh and blood.

"Into Your Hand I Commit My Spirit"

GENERATION AFTER GENERATION THE MOTHERS in Palestine put their children to bed with prayers and soft singing. Jewish mothers in Judea, Galilee, Nazareth, kindly lying on the pallets beside a Yeshi or a Miriam murmured:

"In you, O Lord, we seek refuge ..."

The prayers were a comfort before a deeper darkness and a sleep like death. But as they became familiar songs, they directed and strengthened the trust of the child in the Lord, "My rock and my fortress."

So must Mary have murmured the words over her Jesus at night, the same words whole families sang together as their oil lamps guttered and went out. This prayer, remembered still in Psalm 31:

"Into your hand I commit my spirit; you have redeemed me, O Lord, my faithful God."

And don't our mothers even today do something of the same — use familiar prayers by which to persuade the child that Jesus is always here, even in the dark of sleep, even in the dark of death?

"Now I lay me down to sleep. I pray the Lord my soul to keep. If I should die before I wake, I pray the Lord my soul to take."

Of course. And as long as motherhood continues, so shall that particular consolation.

Now watch what Jesus does on the cross. The infant trust which he learned early remains even unto the end, when the grown man is reduced to infancy again.

The little prayer comes back!

> It was now about noon, and darkness came over the whole land until three in the afternoon, while the sun's light failed. And the curtain of the temple was torn in two. Then Jesus, crying with a loud voice, said: *Father, into your hands I commend my spirit!* Having said this, he breathed his last. (Luke 23)

The trust in his mother's melody (Psalm 31) embraces his whole life, arising again in his "loud voice."

Then, take comfort: as it was with Jesus, so it is with us today. Trust and trustworthiness surround our lives. That which in the beginning granted us an infant peace is here yet again — when we have been returned to helplessness. "Back again," I say, with motherly, fatherly consolation.

If all my life, like Jesus's, is protected by the left hand and the right hand of God, why wouldn't I be able to speak peacefully of this terminal disease?

It is the winter of 1957. An aggressive wind blusters at the eaves of our house. Snow scrolls down the roof, winding into the night. Wind whistles in the plaster-cracks. It is so poorly insulated, this house built before the turn of the century. My attic room receives its little heat from the kitchen through a grate in my floor.

I lie in my bed shivering. Shivering so hard, my muscles ache.

We live in Edmonton, Alberta, Canada.

Though the attic air is, in fact, cold, and the room darkened by these long northern nights, it isn't winter that makes me tremble. It's the fever which suddenly seizes me in my sleep. I dream wildly. In my dreams I am late to class, then sitting naked in the classroom; water is roaring somewhere, silencing the laughter of my classmates. I'm in the water. A mountain stream in the Canadian Rockies. Cold. Finally I come woofing and sweating out of the terrible sleep. Lights pop before my eyes. I try to make sense of my surroundings....

My brother is breathing deeply in another bed, oblivious of my sweating freeze. The wind outside causes an odd, voluminous silence inside. Hollow hallways and empty beds below. In all the house I am the only one awake.

I do not—I will not!—cry or moan privately.

I'm thirteen years old.

Seven months ago, in sweet spring, I stood up before the whole congregation of Bethlehem Church while the pastor examined me regarding the doctrines and teachings of the Christian Faith. My answers were memorized; therefore they were thoughtful, direct, accurate and absolutely true. Moreover, I quoted the Bible to support each answer. My family in the pews bent left and right in order to see me. They smiled their pride at my confirmation.

In that moment I became an adult. Or so it was told me, and I believed it.

An adult: is independent.

An adult: must accomplish things on his own.

An adult: no longer needs the support of his parents. He is in charge. He and Jesus together. Well, *maybe* Jesus. The Lord does not always seem available. Therefore, it is he, this fresh adult, who must perform the deeds.

Something like that. And I've been practicing adulthood ever since.

Therefore, here in my sweat-soaked bed I will not moan nor reveal my weakness to anyone. I do not want to fall back into a whimpering childhood.

But adulthood is so difficult. This lifelong state has become so solitary. I alone am wakeful and watching in the house. If Jesus is really here, I can't see him. Hard, hard to bear so heavy a responsibility. Yet I do not complain. Truly. Even in secret I don't fuss—because this is the way it is for adults. And I am an adult.

Lord! Rock and fortress! My stomach hurts. My stomach is the center of all my sorrows tonight.

I want to bawl.

When we walk outside in this Canadian weather, my hair clicks into an iron cap of ice. All of us, seven children and two parents, crowd into a Volkswagen bus whose only heat blows in from the engine. Dad hunches toward the windshield and rubs the interior frost with his gloved hand, and calls to us: "Breathe through your ears! Breathe through your chins or we'll never get to church!"

He doesn't realize how much my adulthood has excluded me from such silly family customs. They're meant for children.

Now I do begin to cry. A soft snuffling. Just a leaking of my tears. It helps. No, but it doesn't help my soul at all.

Suddenly the heat-grating glows low in the floor. It washes in grey-brown shadows the slants and the angles of my attic ceiling.

Then, a few moments later slender rods of light frame my bedroom door. The door is closed. Now, slowly, it opens. I hold my breath.

There, silhouetted in the doorframe, stands the form of my mother, her nightgown luminous like folded wings. Angels' wings.

I hiccup a sob.

The woman floats into the bedroom, lamplight spilling behind her. She approaches my bed. She sits down on the side of it. No, the woman is not a spirit. She has form and weight. My mattress sags where she sits, and I roll down the incline to the warmth of her thigh.

Finally, helplessly, I lose control. I begin to sob openly, snot chapping my upper lip. But—O dear Jesus—am I permitted such relief?

"Mama?"

In music my mother answers, "I'm here, Wally. I'm right here."

She lays a cool hand on my forehead, then sits in silence awhile.

In the falling light I can see the intelligent expanse of her forehead, the narrow dip of her nose. She bends her head to gaze at me.

"Tell me what's the matter."

"My tummy," I say. It's true. I grab it in both hands. "My tummy."

"Hush, hush." She strokes my hair.

"Here," she says. "Pull your knees up to your chest, and keep them there. You'll fall asleep again. Your stomach will be grateful for the pressure."

I double my legs and draw them up, my kneecaps bumping her on the way. And yes. My mother is right. It helps. Especially when, softly in the winter's night, she begins to sing.

I am an adult at thirteen. I am a child too. Listening to her sweet song, I consider that probably we will *always* be both.

Virginia, my elegant mother, lays her cheek against mine and sings:

I am Jesus' little lamb,
Ever glad at heart I am ...

My brother keeps on sleeping. He knows this song as well as I do. Maybe it's the familiarity that allows him to sleep and still to take the comfort.

The wind diminishes. Its whistling seems to blow an accompaniment. I sing along, though it is my mother's voice that dominates:

For my Shepherd gently guides me,
Knows my need and well provides me ...

THE IMAGE WHICH EVEN NOW most consoles me, as at sixty-four I am given to contemplate another sort of wintry darkness, is that of the Shepherd, and one of the Bible verses memorized for my confirmation examination rises up in me again:

"The sheep hear his voice. He calls his own sheep by name and leads them out."

And again, Jesus himself is speaking:

"My sheep hear my voice. I know them, and they follow me."

There is much more to say about Jesus-the-Shepherd and Wally-the-lamb. Before this volume is finished, we will discover the deeper meaning of these roles, yes, and the genuine peace they bring to our dyings. But for now it is enough to make the following, simpler observation:

Today again, death has uncovered the child in me, the heart filled with childlike longings and an infant's perfect trust.

The song that consoled my earliest years—for Jesus dwelt in the music of my mother—that lullaby comforts me still. Who sings it now? Who carries me now in that sweet chariot with intimacy, grace, and the angels' wings?

My mother's music. The voice of my own spirit, singing along. The companionship of us two and of my wife and my children; the company of faithful friends; the hosts of the heavenly angels—we, all of us, sing a song not different from the song that Jesus sang from the cross:

—for my Shepherd gently guides me,
Knows my need, and well provides me,
Loves me every day the same,
Even calls me by my name.

Day by day, at home, away,
Jesus is my Staff and Stay.
When I hunger, Jesus feeds me,
Into pleasant pastures leads me;
When I thirst, He bids me go
Where the quiet waters flow.

Who so happy as I am,
Even now the Shepherd's lamb?
And when my short life is ended,
By His angel host attended,
He shall fold me to His breast,
There within His arms to rest.

> *Henriette L. von Hayn*
> *in the Brüder Choral-Buch, 1784*

Letters from the Land of Cancer

Part

Letter #1

Monday, January 16, 2006

Friends: I'll tell the thing to you in story form ...

On December 26, while grocery shopping with my grand-daughter Cassindra, I reached up to touch my neck in that hollow just above the left clavicle, where I found a good-sized mass. I can't remember what caused me to lift my hand. Surely no premonition. All my attention was on bread and the beautiful child beside me. Nor do I think I reached to investigate something. An itch. A new sensation. It was a common, unconscious gesture.

But within the instant I realized that I was stroking and measuring a new thing: soft tissue filling the hollow from the clavicular notch back to the beginning of my shoulder. Four inches long? Tucked deeper under the bone than I could feel.

Mildly, I wondered if it were a tumor. Or why else was cushion there? Still pushing the grocery cart, aware of Cassindra ... If it were a tumor, what then?

By good fortune all of our children, their spouses and our grandchildren had gathered at our house for Christmas.

As soon as I'd returned home I took Thanne aside and asked her to touch this thing in my neck. She took it very seriously. We called Dr. Keith Gingerich, our family doctor, and in less than two hours he was examining me. This was a Monday afternoon.

"One of two possibilities," he conjectured. It was a swollen lymph node. Either the node was trying to evacuate an internal infection, or the node was a lymphoma.

Dr. Gingerich didn't hesitate. He sent me directly to Porter Hospital for an X-ray and a CT scan. I went home. Thanne and I said nothing to the others. We didn't know how long we'd have to wait.

As a matter of fact, the very next day I ran into the doctor just outside his offices. He'd asked the radiologist to read the pictures immediately. What usually takes three days had taken but one. We didn't even go into Gingerich's offices. Standing outside in the wintry afternoon, he said, "It looks suspicious. The doctor tells me he's found two other masses in your chest. Likely it's a lymphoma."

That was Tuesday. Wednesday after we had eaten supper, Thanne and I sent away the grandchildren while their parents stayed at the table with Thanne and me. She let me do that talking.

Letter #1

I felt no urgency. It didn't seem as if I were peering into a bleak darkness. Rather, I spoke slowly, choosing my words in order to offer the thing as plainly as possible.

Only one of our four children has never married. Matthew, in his mid-thirties. He lives in Atlanta, Georgia, where he works as the manager of a restaurant. At table on that Wednesday evening he was sitting to my left.

Even as I've written the sequence here for you, so I told it to the children:

Very likely a cancer. In my neck, in the lower part of my left lung, and another underneath my sternum, crossing from lung to lung.

"I'm not afraid," I said to them. "I think of this—whatever is to come, I think of it as an adventure."

In fact, even when I was a pastor sitting with those who were dying, I had begun to characterize my own dying as an "adventure."

"I mean, I'll get to experience things I've never experienced before. It's like traveling to Africa or Japan. Except that this trip will finally leave the world altogether."

I genuinely meant what I was saying. And I meant it to comfort the family. They bent their faces to the table. Catherine, Joseph's wife, gazed directly at me, her eyes steadfast and glittering. Thanne scanned our children to see how they were taking the news. Matt had put his forehead down on the table and covered the back of his neck with his hand.

Perhaps the image didn't have the effect I wanted. Maybe I

made too much of the end of my adventure. Because when we had prayed, when everyone else rose up from the table, Matthew kept his head down, his shoulders hunched.

Then, suddenly, he rose up and walked to the bathroom, shut and locked the door, and there he stayed.

The kitchen was busy. The light bright, dishes cleaned with rubber spatulas, pots and pans rattling. But Matthew didn't come out. Thanne and I looked at each other.

This is the little boy who grew restive whenever I had to be gone from home overnight. More than three nights and Matt could scarcely abide my absence and the brokenness of the family whole.

After about a half hour I knocked on the bathroom door and said, "Matthew, come out. Take a walk with me."

He did. He came out and put on his coat; I, my boots and a thick coat too. The night was cold, the ground dusted with snow.

We walked side by side in silence. The dusk-to-dawn light illumined our going. Thanne and I live in the country.

Finally I talked. "Matt, whatever happens, if ever I have to leave the work to your mother, would you take over?"

He kept his mouth closed. We kept walking.

"You are the most free. You are the best one — the only one — whom I can ask. Will you take care of Mom for me?"

Softly he indicated agreement.

We hugged.

ON FRIDAY OF THAT SAME week, just four days from discovery, Thanne and I met with a chemical oncologist, Dr. Mary Klein.

She wrote an order for a PET scan and then a biopsy by the general surgeon, Dr. Cooper. The PET scan took place soon enough. But I couldn't get an appointment with the surgeon until the following Thursday, January 5. Once he had examined my lump, he scheduled me for surgery the very next day, Friday, January 6, the Feast of the Epiphany. More than a simple biopsy, he removed altogether the mass in my neck.

One week later we returned to Dr. Cooper.

I have, he told us, a metastatic cancer. That is, the cancers in my lymph nodes are not the primary source. They've metastasized from somewhere else in my body, most probably from the littlest tumor in my left lung.

THIS AFTERNOON, THE 16TH, THANNE and I will drive to Chesterton to meet with Dr. Klein again. She'll talk about therapies. We have already (well, Thanne has) called the children to let them know what we know.

To add to the complications: I've just had four molars surgically removed. Dr. Lisa Shideler tells me that she can often sense the presence of a cancer before others know it, because trouble with teeth seems to be symptomatic. The molars had to be removed before anything like chemotherapy or radiation or my lowered white cell blood count might permit new infections. Chewing has become an acrobatic twisting of the tongue.

OKAY. THIS IS WHERE WE are right now. All these things are harder on Thanne than they are on me. Her waiting and the weight upon her shoulders outreaches mine. And those who don't have the disease yearn deeply to take it from their beloved — but they can't. They can only watch.

I promise you, I am at peace. We have a wonderful community surrounding us here in Valparaiso, both the town and our church and the university. And my faith, despite so much I do not know, looks forward to the Kingdom.

Peace. Peace to all of you. There is little enough of peace in the world right now. Let it be, then, in our hearts. We are not of the world. We are of the angels who wished peace upon everyone when the Messiah was born.

Walt

Letter # 2

IT'S THE LAST MONDAY OF January. I'm in my university office
—about a half hour before I meet with a blessed gathering of
writing students, all of us doing this exercise once a week, Mondays. A Master's Class, since these have already taken my seminar
in creative writing—the exit course for majors and minors.

We discuss the writing of their previous week, doing this
thing for the pleasure of it, neither for money nor for credit. I love
to teach. I love these students, their tenderness and their produce.
Creative writers often seem odd to their classmates, the major-
ity of young undergraduates who see *them*selves as a cut above
the common, and who are comforted in their mutual affirma-
tions. But these my artists' ("weird") characteristics have already

31

granted them sharp insight, the somewhat solitary practice of self-exploration, and the steadfast, perceptive observation of the world, that cyclorama encircling the whole of each.

I tell them of my own experience, how "weird" I've felt too, and how separated all my life long. How that the abused child learns early to read the faces of others, seeking to know the mood even before that more powerful other knows her own mood and acts on it. Such a child shapes and reshapes himself, enacts desperate games to escape another round of pain. As he grows, his self-uncertainty defines him as "different." But his penetrating vision, reading in external details the internal meanings, finally empowers him after all.

"Rather than suffer society's scorn, use your sight/insight as your advantage over society."

Already now, a day before my first chemotherapeutic session, people who know of my cancer have repeated well-meant formulas in such a way as to indicate a slight distance between themselves and me.

Well, what can you say to someone who has a killing disease? Especially when you're not practiced at the conversation—and when you yourself feel the difference, as if the one afflicted has been removed from the common life and a kind of cellophane wraps him away?

Even so (just over a month from the days of my diagnosis) do I put myself in the shoes of those who feel unable to put themselves in mine.

LET THIS BE MY SECOND personal update regarding the things that have chosen to grow inside my body (things, I must confess, which are themselves parts of my body, supported by my blood and my own oxygen, of the same substance, if not of the same structure, as other body parts. Interesting. It actually plays havoc with one of the paradigms so many people are urging me to accept: to FIGHT).

"It comes of the devil!" one elderly woman admonished me with intensity. This was on a Sunday when I had preached in the University Chapel. She narrowed her eye and uttered, prophetlike: "Overcome him! The victory of Jesus! Pray the evil spirits out!"

My cancer has been calculated as stage IIIB. There are four stages altogether, measured against at least three grids of diagnosis. The "stage" suggests the sort of therapy most necessary. In my case — the cancer's having metastasized from a tumor (about 3 centimeters small) in my left lung into two other masses involving large clutches of lymph nodes both in my neck and in my chest, and that third tumor's having spread across the medial region of my sternum — I am diagnosed nearer the top of the four stages than the bottom. (O ye medical personnel who happen to find this letter, forgive me my ignorance of oncological terms and procedures. I'm a neophyte, only just learning. *What* three grids?)

But this I do know by the anticipation of the experience: my stage requires a most aggressive response. I will undergo two oncological therapies at once: chemotherapy and radiation therapy. Chemo is once a week, Tuesdays. Radiation is every week day, Mondays through Fridays, usually at four in the afternoon.

Walt

Letter #3

Friends:

It's Tuesday now, the last day in January.

I'm sitting in a deep-cushioned reclining chair (too soft; these flop-chairs break my back) the drip-tube attached to a port in my chest, running poisons through my bloodstream in order to save me alive. The poisons are meant to heal me. What ironies, hey?

I'm writing to you as I sit. It passes the time. Better, it *redeems* the time of my physical captivity, conjuring your spirits here. Well, and I'll be sitting here approximately two and a half hours — or three, depending on today's reaction. The first fluid administered through the tube and into my chest (about an hour ago) prepared my body safely to accept the water-clear poisons now flooding my system. That initial infusion seems to have worked because of the whopping amount of Benadryl it contained.

Last week, however—Tuesday, January 24, when I sat here for my first chemical therapy—an allergic reaction interrupted the process. The flesh of my face was set afire. My breathing grew constricted, as if the ribs were clamping closed my lungs. My heart rate shot into my throat. I felt a desperate kind of thrill at the toboggan-drop of my bodily functions.

Soon enough the technicians cut off the chemicals and introduced a saline drip. Next they filled the plastic sack with another dose of Benadryl. In less than half an hour the trouble passed.

Now, among a number of elderly people—women whose scarves cover their bald heads; men cranked backward in their easy chairs, snoring; some people reading; some watching *Jeopardy* on TV—I crouch forward and write, drawing your company into my little room.

My symptoms.

Or, rather, the more evident manifestations of all this to-ing and fro-ing between tumors and physicians, between organic and technological forces:

Not bad. My hair is still in the root. If it will fall out, I understand that the loss won't begin till after the late second or the third week of these therapies—though when and whether seems to depend upon each individual's physiological characteristics.

My swallow, my bread-basket, my guts—those elastic sausage casings—feel as if I, like the chicken, had pecked and ingested gravel. Gravel in me does not stop at the gizzard. It travels and scratches right through the softer parts.

On the other hand, nowadays there are medications that help us (patients) keep our food down. Nausea doesn't wrack us so much anymore. I don't throw up, though the mass in my neck seems to press against the throat, causing sensations of thick mucous globs hanging near my gag-reflex and these I can't hack up and out.

I grow tired quickly. Headaches.

Dr. Klein ordered a brain scan. "Don't worry," saying to me. "We need a baseline reading against which to measure any changes." Changes? I'm told that after a while this weariness will increase until it becomes a constant exhaustion — a cumulative progression — and that I may indeed experience greater and greater distress in swallowing.

I'm ready.

I'm still teaching and writing. I had to cancel a trip to New York, though, where a musical based on *The Book of the Dun Cow* is even now in the midst of its tech week. By the time I'm back in this chair again, it will be up and running offffff Broadway. I was scheduled to play the Narrator's role for the first several performances. But therapies and masses have intervened. And, in fact, I don't mind — however great the pleasure I would have taken in a New York applause.

Still mentoring writers: I genuinely love the students whom I am privileged to teach here at Valpo. Every year a new community is formed of new seniors and myself. It has taken a good long while, but finally I've learned how to perform this elemental trick, teaching.

If everything goes well, my therapy will last through seven weeks. We'll take pictures and measurements at the half to watch whether bad things are increasing. Then, at the end of the series, we will search my wounds.

"To search one's wounds." Consider the grace and the mystic service in that phrase. In Malory's *Morte d'Arthur*, as the fellowship of the round table is descending into fractiousness and failure — its twilight deepening — the knights all gather one last time in sad community. They know that such a communion will never come again. But the good Sir Urry lies sick of seven wounds at King Arthur's court. Every knight handles Urry's wounds, by courtesy and loyalty, by goodness and faith and the love of God trying to heal him. One by one they come. But all of them fail. In fact, Sir Urry's wounds open at every new touching and bleed again. Finally, all the knights prayed Sir Launcelot to search his wounds. "Devoutly kneeling, Launcelot ransacked the wounds that bled a little, and forthwith the wounds fair healed and seemed as they had been whole a seven year." Love and melancholy at the loss of love shadow the spirits of Arthur's fellowship. They shall never meet in healing again.

I confess it. Though scarcely spoken and hidden in my bowels, something of that terrible mercy and its sad conclusion accompanies the searching of my wounds in the weeks to come. Will the hands of my own communion heal me? Or what? Will the wounds open like mouths to consume me by parts?

So then, the searching: CT scans, PET scans, MRIs, three times a week the drawing of my blood. We will compare progressively the pictures of innards revealed.

NONETHELESS! IN SPITE OF THE paradox this must pose, I repeat what I've written before: I am completely at peace with this drama. This adventure. Even the seeming of my body's loss—that swift invasion of allergenic symptoms caused by the chemicals last week—hasn't stolen from me the blessings of my adventure.

God does not cause human misery, nor does he desire the death of any person on earth. But he can and does participate in the complexities of human life. He takes, therefore, advantage of our weaknesses to love our spirits and to prop up our weary bones.

That all our children with their families should (unplanned) have gathered at our house this Christmas; that it should have been in those same days that Thanne and I discovered the cancer, so that we might communicate right at the beginning my diagnosis; that I am surrounded with such wonderful students, dear, fierce, cynical and sweetly beloving—all these conjunctions smack of the divine.

Healing is surely to come. It may be the healing of my body. I expect so with all my heart. Or it may be the healing of my weary spirit, which has not *always* been peaceful in the run and the muck, the thistles and the sweats of this worldly existence. This last rest I do also expect with all my heart. I won't be surprised to hear the voice of the Lord at the end of things physical. I believe in both. It is not reasonable. Even to myself I cannot make these pieces fit. A paradox. No, greater: a mystery.

"I saw Satan fall like lightning from heaven," says the Savior. "But don't rejoice in this, that the spirits submit to you, but rejoice that your names are written in the book of heaven." My name. The Father who named me at my Baptism will in a creating and re-creating voice call my name once more, and I shall arise, and I shall like Moses answer, "Here I am."

FRIDAY, JUST FOUR DAYS AGO, I lectured to, I don't know, about sixty people—a kindly gathering, attentive, all sitting in folding chairs. I mentioned my cancer. I followed that thought with a brief description of the surgical procedure by which a port was implanted under the flesh of the right side of my chest, about four inches above the nipple. Having said that, spontaneously, I asked how many of the audience had (or had had) ports like mine. Some twelve hands went up. All women.

Ah, company! I have joined the congregation of the wounded.

Walt

A First Meditation: "Remember, Mortal!"

······

WE HAD JUST BURIED PHYLLIS's father. The death had not been sudden. He had been an elderly gentleman, failing for a while, then dying neither in pain nor in disgrace.

Nor had Phyllis broken into open tears during the funeral service or at the interment. Her grieving had been modest. I admired the dignity of her dress and her comportment.

After the other mourners had left the cemetery, I stood beside the woman awhile. She laid a pale rose on the cylinder hump of the coffin. Phyllis Falk: her fingernails were as translucent as the skin of her fingers, making the nails almost invisible. Her blonde hair, blue eyes, and closed, foreshortened mouth caused me to think of Shirley Temple, but gaunt and world-weary.

Finally the attendants couldn't stall their duties any more.

Phyllis and I watched them crank the casket and her father down to the bottom of the hole. She held a hanky to her nose.

I asked whether I could give her a ride home. Foolish question. What else would she have done? I don't remember why she was left alone. Where had Bernie gone — her husband of eighteen years? Well, maybe he expected the low, black Cadillac that had brought Phyllis to take her back to the church at least. But even the funeral car had departed without her.

She said yes.

I had a green Volkswagen bug. Only a slim space between us. I drove soberly into the city, and slower than the speed limits. Halfway home, I turned onto Division Street. All along the side of that street was a row of small shops. This was a Saturday.

Suddenly Phyllis slapped the windshield and screamed.

I looked over. Her face was enraged: the back of her neck blotched a furious red. She was glaring out at the shops.

"Phyllis! What's wrong?"

"Those people!" she cried. "Those people!"

Yes. There were a few people walking the sidewalk with shopping bags.

"How can they just … go about their lives like that? How can they walk into stores and buy things and walk out of stores *as if nothing's happened?*"

I began to understand. I didn't blame her anger.

Mighty God, the world had just cracked. In *her* world (but to her that *was* the world). From the grave, through the city, a fissure was splitting the ground beneath her feet.

41

How could her father's death *not* toll the great blue bell of the skies? Nothing would ever be the same again. Why didn't these people stop and cover their mouths, subdued?

Her daddy had died.

Her life had been interrupted by death.

All things, all things on this natural earth had been shaken and changed forever.

Suddenly — in the midst of a life fresh and green and full of dreams — death intrudes. Your death. The real thing. *Das ding an sich*, as the Germans say: "The thing itself."

And what may in the past have been a warning, perhaps a multitude of warnings, has suddenly become a dead-eyed decree. No longer is it the caution, "You will die." Now it is the absolute mandate: "You *are* dying."

And with that sentence comes "the dread of something after death, / The undiscovered country from whose bourn / No traveler returns."

"Thus says the Lord: 'Set your house in order, for you shall die. You shall not recover.'"

Oh, God! My God! What is left for me?

"My flesh," shouts Job, stunned into the recognition that no consolation can serve him any more. Neither wealth nor status nor a good family nor even his personal righteousness protects against The Ending. "My flesh," Job cries out, "is clothed with worms and dirt" — his flesh *is* a cloak of worms feeding upon the dirt of his corpus — "my days are swifter than a weaver's shuttle, and come to their end without hope."

Set your house in order!

When these are our conditions and our attitudes, when we remain unprepared for the Ultimatum certainly to seize us, then the death that interrupts our daily lives is monstrous. Fight against it with all your might. Hate it. Be filled with envy and anger for those who are still healthy. Wail, plead, beg, make deals with friends and with the Infinite. Sink into despair. Lie down in hopelessness. Die, then — even before you die.

Or else, prepare. Long before that final confrontation, prepare.

HERMAN THOMAS TELLS ME THE story of his father's passage into death.

Herman is a member of Grace Church where I spent nearly fifteen years as its pastor. African American, central city, independent, profoundly humble, profoundly dignified, deeply faithful, the members of Grace bore me up more than I did them.

I knew his father finally as a gaunt man, stringy and slightly bowed in the shoulders. His head was smaller than his son's, his complexion not so rich and dark — a little powdered, it seemed, by a layer of sickness.

"I sat with him, Pastor. This day and the next one. He lay still. Straight up and down on the sheets. Didn't say the first word. But I hummed. Kept it soft. Hummed in my nose. And I stroked his little hair. And didn't matter if I sat in a hospital or else a house, 'cause Daddy made the room his bedroom and whatever the building, a home."

Herman is a short, placid man. He sits with his hands fitted each to a knee. When he stands he's no higher than my nose. Because of the earnestness of his messages, he raises his eyebrows when he speaks, puckers his forehead and widens his eyes. His expression is meant to convey assurance: *Yes, yes, this is true and very important.* Yet his natural smile gentles the persuasion.

"And then it was a shadowy afternoon when he came to die. Pastor, Daddy opened his eyes. His eyes roved around the room. Left and right without a turn of his head. Down and up. Then he picked out a high corner of the ceiling, up and off to his right."

Herman's sight goes inward. He is nodding, and all his features are softening.

"He never took his eyes down from that corner. He reached and took my arm. And then he talked. After days, the first time he talked.

"Daddy said, 'Herman, you can't see her. I'm sorry you can't see her. But there's Mama. She's waiting for me.'"

Soon thereafter, a man of no complaint, fully trusting in the light of Jesus, closed his eyes again and died.

Nor did his son take sorrow from the scene.

Immanuel.

"It was Jesus took him to the heaven of my Mama and his wife."

It's evening. All the church lights muted. People move forward from their pews to the railing around the altar. They kneel. They fold their hands and bow their heads.

A pastor meets every one of the worshippers who kneel before him. He places his hands on each bowed head and bends low in order to murmur to that one alone.

"Memento, homo," he says: *"Quia pulvis es, et in pulverem reverteris."*

The pastor turns to an assistant who carries a small metal box of ashes. Into this he dips his finger. Then, turning back to the worshipper, he draws in black two small lines, each intersecting the other. This is the cross which she shall wear out of the church and into the world again — the cross in the midst of her daily life. Here is a sign of Christ's death, into which by his grace we may ourselves die. Here too, if we would accept it, is the sign of our own final dying, the death at the ends of our lives. And see? They have been made one. What have I to fear?

"Remember, mortal," the pastor murmurs, defining the sign, expressing our need for the crucified Savior: "Remember: you are dust and to dust you shall return."

This is Ash Wednesday. This is the ritual which my worship tradition has repeated year after year after year, allowing the cross to appear on our foreheads in private and in public.

How mournful. Oh, how depressing, do you say?

Perhaps. I won't argue the mood of the moment.

But I rejoice in its effect! For this is one way by which the church calls Christians to "remember" what is to come; to awaken even now to the End ("for night is flying"); to contemplate each his and her own iniquities and therefore to repent; to see and to believe that we shall, when we die, die into Christ's victorious death — and so to hope.

All of which, you see, is to prepare.

MORE TIMES THAN I CAN count, I've spoken the following words by the graves of members of my congregation.

Phyllis's father lies in his shining casket which, under a floral bouquet, lies on the straps and the structure by which he will be lowered into the sheer pit below.

But first we must acknowledge this death—and therein, our deaths too.

The words I speak are meant to comfort Phyllis and the mourners gathered around the grave with us. Wind flaps the edges of our canopy. A whirling rain causes people to duck deeper into their coats. In order for all to hear me, I have to raise my voice.

Whether they are meant to or not, they change my soul, these words, enlarging my sense of death and, therefore, enlarging my sense of life. Because I must say them so often, because I say them in the heat of crises and certain emotions, they drive as deep as roots into me.

I've said them when there were no more than three of us beside a tiny hole in the ground. Three: myself, the mother of a stillborn child, and the child in a white casket so small I have carried it in two hands.

I've repeated exactly the same words for the young man shot to death by other young men. No reason. Mistaken identity.

And for the old, and for the well-diseased, and for the deeply weary—so often, they have prepared also me to receive the news of my lung cancer without horror, without some other hopeless mortification. But with a certain valid equanimity:

A First Meditation: "Remember, Mortal!"

Forasmuch as it hath pleased Almighty God,
in his wise providence,
to take out of this world the soul of our departed brother,
we therefore commit his body to the ground;
earth to earth, ashes to ashes, dust to dust:
in the hope of the resurrection to eternal life,
through our Lord Jesus Christ,
who shall change our vile body
that it may be fashioned like unto his glorious body,
according to the working whereby he is able
even to subdue all things unto himself.

May God the Father,
    who has created this body;
May God the Son,
    who by his blood has redeemed this body together with the soul;
May God the Holy Spirit,
    who by baptism has sanctified this body to be his temple—
    keep these remains unto the day of the resurrection of all flesh.
Amen.

Letter #4

March 6, 2006

Friends:

It's snowing. It's Sunday. The snowfall began near noon and has continued since then, now into the evening. Into the gloaming, as it seems to me. The air is dimensioned by the feathering fall of the flakes, swiftly down nearby, slowly down afar. But it does not altogether blank the fields and the trees outside. I can see as through a bridal veil.

The temperature hovers below 30 degrees, so each small flake makes a "tick" against my window. I've just come back from walking outside.

I took my time. Lately I lose my breath so quickly. In the

afternoons or the evenings I find myself exhausted, falling asleep in a blink, to wake on the sofa, in bed and finally sleeping fitfully.

But I need the exercise, so I walk a dozen paces ascending a low rise, and pause to breathe, sucking oxygen back into the blood.

We have woods on our land, Thanne and I. The tracks of many creatures show me how busy things are outside. Through the ghosts of such business I move: deer tracks, the toes of their hooves scoring the snows; rabbit tracks bunching in tight groups of four; the neat hands of raccoons, tiny flits of mice. I envy them. They don't have trouble traveling. But all is silent during my snowy walk. Breath-holes tunnel down to a groundhog's burrow.

Breathlessness. Singing hymns takes my breath away. My voice has deepened to a genuine bass. Higher notes cause me to cough. I cannot finish two lines of a hymn without having to sit down, puffing.

So these are the things on my mind these days: that I must spend slow time moving through the drifts — not only for the exercise after all. I go for the beauty and the silent intimacy of the going. I go without any morbidity whatsoever. I think: *Maybe this is my last opportunity to walk in a winter's snowfall.* Not to make a memory of it, but to know it now. I don't mind that I have to take my time.

Let's see if I can explain.

It's often said that once one confronts an imminent death, he/she changes, thereafter striving to experience each day to the fullest. Every moment — so goes the conventional talk — must become a lifetime. Intense awareness, a drilling focus on things present, a hasty cramming of sensations tries to make up for all the past years of dumb, numb neglect. Why had they spent all those previous years rushing into tomorrow? It is because of the sudden brevity of the rest of their lives that they grow greedy for the Now. Well, and the Now might, in fact, shut off melancholy meditations upon this loss of so much goodness when they still had so many years before. These final days must more than balance the rest. These final days have become their lifetimes whole.

Nor do I doubt that this talk might be a generalized description of another's response to a terminal illness.

But in my case it seems much simpler. I find that I just pay attention.

However short or long my personal journey hereafter (a year, years, or half a year) time present remains for me what it always was before: an opportunity to pay attention. Time doesn't become more intense. Time is … time. I am now. It is enough.

I have always loved to walk in the woods and to work our land. And because of the wheeling seasons, no walk is the same as another. Work around here changes old to new, in obedience to the seasons. But that *is* what time has been and still continues to be: variety winter and spring, yesterday and tomorrow. An adventure walking, working. The difference between my past and my present — having begun to bear a cancer inside my body — is no more than this, I take again the same opportunity as always, but possibly now for the last time.

If I sought a greater intensity than what is, well, that would only take my breath away more often, and my ability to pay attention would be too much curtailed.

Is this too much interior contemplation? Sorry. Here's information more concrete.

My radiation continues apace. I'm about halfway through the series. I think they planned thirty-seven treatments. I've had a little over twenty. After we've run this race to the end, there will be another week of spot-shots. The doctor tells me that two of the masses have been reduced by my treatments heretofore. His figures are estimates, but he says of the tumor central in my chest that it has shrunk from five centimeters to three. Radiation now causes what they call "discomfort" in my chest and abdomen. (I liken that word "discomfort" to the words "you'll feel a little pinch" before the needle bites my skin with the fire of a wasp-sting and the burning afterward.)

But the pain enclosed in my torso is like the intrusion of a sapling inside of me, roots in the lower guts, twigs in my throat—something to keep me awake at nights.

The chemotherapy has been somewhat bumpier. My blood counts have dropped too often too low. Two times now the diminishing of white cells has made any therapy too dangerous—and if it should go any lower, we'll have to suspend the radiation treatments. For now the oncologist has ordered for me the biweekly injection of another sort of chemical, this to increase the production of white cells in the marrow of my larger bones. It seems to be working. That's good. But those larger bones have set up an unhappy complaining. They ache. The new chemical has whacked them, causing in me the sensation of a deep, deep bruising—and still my platelets are too low. Soon I'll receive the chemo treatments at half dosage every other week and see what happens. This will extend the weeks of these therapies.

Your letters, my friends, your expressions of support and companionship have been for me a blessed conversation. And the varieties of your thoughts have made of the conversation a community of fine complexity. I mean: it has been for me—without my moving from my home—a dear pleasure.

The pole-light outside the house is making a cone of snowfall in the darkness. It's getting colder outside. The flakes are tighter, smaller. Ticking sounds like fingernails drumming the window glass.

How good to have good friends! Goodnight.

Walt

A Second Meditation: Rinsed with Gold, Endless, Walking the Fields

...·...

As for the glory of the natural world, the creation into which the Lord God has placed us, read the following hymn written by my friend, the poet Robert Siegel.

> *Let this day's air praise the Lord—*
> *Rinsed with gold, endless, walking the fields,*
> *Blue and bearing the clouds like censers,*
> *Holding the sun like a single note*
> *Running through all things, a basso profundo*
> *Rousing the birds to an endless chorus.*
>
> *Let the river throw itself down before him,*
> *The rapids laugh and flash with his praise,*

Let the lake tremble about its edges
And gather itself in one clear thought
To mirror the heavens and the reckless gulls
That swoop and rise on its glittering shores.

Let the lawn burn continually before him
A green flame, and the tree's shadow
Sweep over it like the baton of a conductor,
Let the winds hug the housecorners and woodsmoke
Sweeten the world with her invisible dress,
Let the cricket wind his heartspring
And draw the night by like a child's toy.

Let the tree stand and thoughtfully consider
His presence as its leaves dip and row
The long sea of winds, as sun and moon
Unfurl and decline like contending flags.

Let the blackbirds quick as knives praise the Lord,
Let the sparrow line the moon for her nest
And pick the early sun for her cherry,
Let her slide on the outgoing breath of evening,
Telling of raven and dove,
The quick flutters, homings to the green houses.

Let the worm climb a winding stair,
Let the mole offer no sad explanation
As he paddles aside the dark from his nose,
Let the dog tug on the leash of his bark,

The startled cat electrically hiss,
And the snake sign her name in the dust

In joy. For it is he who underlies
The rock from its liquid foundation,
The sharp contraries of the giddy atom,
The unimaginable curve of space,
Time pulling like a patient string,
And gravity, fiercest of natural loves.

At his laughter, splendor riddles the night,
Galaxies swarm from a secret hive,
Mountains lift their heads from the sea,
Continents split and crawl for aeons
To huddle again, and planets melt
In the last tantrum of a dying star.

At his least signal spring shifts
Its green patina over half the earth,
Deserts whisper themselves over cities,
Polar caps widen and wither like flowers.

In his stillness rock shifts, root probes,
The spider tenses her geometrical ego,
The larva dreams in the heart of the peachwood,
The child's pencil makes a shaky line,
The dog sighs and settles deeper,
And a smile takes hold like the feet of a bird.

Sit straight, let the air ride down your backbone,
Let your lungs unfold like a field of roses,
Your eyes hang the sun and moon between them,
Your hands weigh the sky in even balance,
Your tongue, swiftest of members, release a word
Spoken at the conception to the sanctum of genes,
And each breath rise sinuous with praise.

Let your feet move to the rhythm of your pulse
(Your joints like pearls and rubies he has hidden),
And your hands float high on the tide of your feelings.
Now, shout from the stomach, hoarse with music,
Give gladness and joy back to the Lord,
Who, sly as a milkweed, takes root in your heart.

   From In a Pig's Eye: Poems
    by Robert Siegel

Letter #5

March 26, 2006

Dear Friends:

They keep the TV on in this room. I've never seen it off. My chemo appointments begin at a quarter past one in the afternoon. Game shows, soap operas, talk shows. Only newcomers actually pay attention. Regular patients allow their eyes to settle on the screen. Because it's a focus of color and motion and sound, I think. But there's a sprightly, kerchiefed, painfully thin lady sitting at an angle from me who is reading. Novels. When she has finished one, she leaves it behind for others to read—though I haven't noticed that anyone else ever picks one up and reads what she has graciously offered.

Some of my neighbors knit. Most of the old men doze. A

young man (but he comes less frequently than I do) works furiously at a laptop. Me too. Right now I've got my laptop open on my lap, and I'm crouched forward, pecking the keys and writing to you.

Please: if these letters become repetitive or morbid or long and dull for you, I must believe in your freedom to toss them. Then I shan't be troubled by laying on you burdens you wouldn't wish to bear.

The first series of radiation therapy came to an end yesterday. This ought to kick the chemotherapy—as the Bam! chef says—"up a notch," or two or three. I've asked my doctors to be as aggressive as they safely can be. Certainly I'll be receiving bites from the head of this plastic serpent weekly, now; perhaps its tooth will also spit into me the full dose each time.

Two Sundays now I've worshipped with several of our grandchildren. Noah and Emma. Daughter Mary has come to help Thanne paint walls in the house. This is a labor beyond me. I can scarcely climb steps. But another labor ... we have considered it necessary that I interact with the grandkids rather more than is usual for me. Well, you know. What time is left? And how will they remember me after this?

In church, upon a whim, I asked Emma (kindergarten) whether I could look at her hand. She gave it to me, her left hand in my right, and without question allowed me to keep it a full ten minutes.

Oh, the exercise moved me! I watched the thin blue veins in

her wrist. Press in a certain place, and one vein vanishes. I studied the hangnails, the uneven edges of the fingernails themselves, the back of her hand. Her palm. I've never done this before. It made the moment, and even the worship, very intimate for me: no self-consciousness on Emma's part. She scarcely looked at her Papa looking at her. How lovely such a trust.

To see the small things, to look more closely at her milk-white hand, I have to put my glasses up on my forehead and move inches away and peer intently down. That was just fine with Emma. And something filled me with consolation; for to know her hand in such focused detail, the thing she puts daily to a thousand uses, wherewith she touches and caresses and grabs and slaps and signals and pets the dog and writes and points to the words she's reading — to know her hand is to approach her soul.

Remember me.

After Emma, Noah.

In church he's more squirrelly than his sister and generally more demanding. He insists on questioning the things that happen around him and to him.

Nevertheless, Noah took my request, and then my holding of his hand upside-up and downside-up, took my near peering at his knuckles all in stride. His nails have a shape distinctly different from Emma's: broader, tougher. He has fewer hangnails. And though his wrist is not much larger — a willow-slender wrist, scarcely capable of doing heavy work — he is capable of doing the work anyway. You know: throwing a ball hard. Pulling a black greyhound named Magic. Cracking solid objects in sudden rushes of anger. Upon the skin of the hands of both my grand-children I could find no hair. That's for yet-to-come, even while my loss of hair happens for me.

I will examine the hands of all my grandchildren before I'm through. We'll see how peacefully each one accepts the grandfa-therly intrusion. I can imagine that one of them, Maxwell, might not have the patience. But Noah surprised me. Max may too.

PAINTING THE HOUSE. THE LAST week or two of radiation has simply exhausted me. And when I stand or cough hard, I sense a serious dislocation. I mean that (like dizziness, but not quite diz-ziness itself) the world around me resolves itself into something like a movie, a film for which I am the audience, neither actor nor participant.

But this baffles me. No, it doesn't: for important purposes I can husband my strength. This previous Sunday I preached for two services in the Chapel of the Resurrection. One can almost measure the amount of energy in one's tank; so I sat while others stood; and I sat on a stool through most of my sermons; I didn't shake hands at the end of the service (Thanne warns me: "Too many people with too many germs!")—and so I could accom-plish the task after all. I am scheduled to preach again on Easter Sunday. I look forward to that assignment. Christ the Lord is risen again!

My father, the year of his retirement, received not one invi-tation to preach on Easter. He called me that afternoon. "I'm dying, Wally," he said to me, "dying." For him this was not a metaphor.

THERE WAS A PERIOD — perhaps ten days long, perhaps two weeks — when I began to handle things bitingly.

This is a confession, and necessary.

I lost serenity, patience, goodness with regard to other people. I grew high-handed with various nurses, the nurse-practitioners, the technicians who conduct my therapies or take my blood, those who take internal looks into my vitals by CT scans — and with the gatekeepers to all these places.

The elderly woman who volunteers to organize the many patients who come to the clinic for their scans — she does me no harm. But I have often gone through her waiting room to meet my appointment. This time she stopped me and shocked me thereby. She wanted me to register first. How self-centered! I'm the one who's sick!

I make my ill-will known not by shouting, but by lowering my voice to a murmurous level, partly to make a show of my admirable self-restraint, partly to menace these supercilious people. I speak in a dense and complex grammar with a ten-dollar vocabulary. And I gaze directly into my interlocutor's eyes. Haughtiness can reduce another to servitude, unless it is ignored. It is powerful. It is wrong.

Thanne and I are clear that if people outside our immediate family require of us strong assurances and consolations, we are not beholden. We've enough to do confronting our diminished and pressing circumstances right here in our own home. We must first spend our spiritual energies on children and grandchildren.

But this does not give me the right to trouble people who are my professional helpers, or people who have no idea of my condition. And when I weigh the different effects upon my soul—meeting people with kindness against meeting people grudgingly and with a peremptory attitude—I find that the latter is hugely more taxing.

And before God, it is wrong.

The elderly volunteer in the clinic responded tit for tat. She grew as snappish with me as I had been with her. So maybe I didn't humiliate her after all. But I stole something of the goodness of her day.

Who tells me that a terminal sickness gives me the right? That folks must meet *me* with understanding?

Under Christ, whose greatest anguishes are delineated in the Gospels by writers at pains to persuade his followers that he met it all without sarcasm or criticism or a self-centered complaint, but met it with serenity and forgiveness, with grace and a genuine love for the world that was even then dispatching him—under Christ my pettiness is wrong.

Well, and that is the word and the generosity I want after all: "Grace."

I beg God that I might do this thing with grace and gracefully, no matter its length or its ending.

Letter #5

DEAR FRIENDS, I DELIGHT IN your longish letters, your blessed, wandering thoughts, your willingness to allow me into your lives these days. Every such communication is like a visit to me, and I take the time to read your sentences and sentiments, and the odd turns your thinking takes. You are not making work for me with these epistles. You are surrounding me with community.

All sincerely,

Walt

A Third Meditation: Noah Insists on Questioning Things

. . . . . .

WHEN HE WAS ABOUT FOUR years old, Noah and I went walking through the acreage behind our house. The grass had not been mown. It stood as high as his waist. I stomped a path to ease his going.

Near the back of the field, shortly before the edge of our woodlands, we both noticed two tall brown stalks above the sweeping level of the grass. We paused, then went more slowly forward.

The stalks turned out to be the ears of a brown doe, who rose up and stood facing us, those ears like radar dishes cupped for sound. We kept moving. The deer took a half-jump away, stopped to stare a moment longer, then sailed gracefully into the trees.

Hidden, she made the vocalized huffing sound of command (or fear). Immediately two smaller heads popped up over the grass. Fawns, stretching their necks but not getting up.

I stopped, but Noah kept moving closer and closer to the fawns. He crouched as he went. As happens when the boy becomes excited, his own large ears grew red, his hair shone ruddy with fresh sweat above the grasses. He began to giggle softly.

It was astonishing to me how close the fawns allowed the boy to approach. Their mother increased her huffing, but they seemed fascinated by the pink cub closing in. He was but ten steps away when one after the other they humped up their rumps and stood—again, just looking at him. His giggling threatened them not a bit.

When they did take to the air to join their mother, Noah laughed aloud and dropped to the ground grabbing his tummy with unspeakable pleasure.

SINCE HE IS THE OLDEST of all our grandchildren, he was the first I took into our woods to camp with me.

This was approximately one year later.

We had already pitched the tent, unrolled our sleeping bags, and eaten several sandwiches by the time we sallied forth to scout the forest floor in the light of the late afternoon. It was my plan to show him the various dens of forest creatures, groundhogs, squirrels, rabbits, foxes. There were black raspberries in the clearings. Possums, raccoons. We were sure to see something.

And we did.

Noah snuck ahead of me, eager and perfectly fearless. Ahead I saw shafts of an angled sunlight splashing leaf mold in an open space. So did Noah see the illuminated ground—and something else as well. For suddenly he crouched down. He began to spit-giggle and bore himself like a small coyote forward.

"Papa."

"What is it?"

"Papa! A deer."

Behind him I pinched my eyesight in order to see the better. Yes: a deer lying motionless on its side, as if melting into the darker ground.

"Noah, wait."

He didn't wait. So I rushed ahead to catch him, careless of the racket I made.

The head of this deer had been thrown so far backward its skull pressed against its withers. From its abdomen there seemed to flow a slow fall of thickened water, ivory-white, rippling in the golden sunlight.

There was such a stench around the deer that I fought a gag. Noah, though, was merely attentive, standing very still, now that I had caught up with him.

"Papa," pointing to that ivory flow, "what's that?"

I told him. I said, "Maggots, Noah. Hundreds of thousands of maggots. They come from the hundreds of thousands of eggs that flies laid on the deer's insides. They are turning the deer into dirt again."

LATER, WHILE WE LAY IN the tent, Noah suddenly spoke out of the darkness. He hadn't gone to sleep.

"Papa?"

"Noah?"

"What was that?—what we saw in the woods."

"I told you already. Little tiny worms, all doing their job, chomp, chomp, chomp." *Ashes to ashes, dust to dust.* But a grandpa can make a joke of it, right?

"No, what was the deer?" Noah's question was solemn but strange.

"A deer. Just a deer. What do you mean?"

"He was sick."

I said, "No, Noah. That deer was dead."

"Ohhh. Then what is 'dead'?"

Ah, Noah! The minds of little children cannot be big enough to hold the heavier lessons of life, can they?

"Did you see the deer's eyes?"

"Yes. No."

He was right. The eyeballs had been plucked away.

"That is dead. No thinking any more. No brains, no breathing, no spirit inside the body of the deer. Only just the body is left."

We lay in silence then a good long while. I thought my grandson had slipped away in sleep.

But he hadn't. He had one more question.

"Papa?"

"What?"

"Can a papa be a dead one too?"

Letter #6

A Letter Never Sent

FIVE MONTHS AGO I BOUGHT a 2006 Ridgeline by Honda. The truck was new. Red. Maybe the last vehicle I'll buy—or so I intend. Intended.

Last week I tore it up in an accident. My fault.

I had turned right on a red light. The traffic east on Highway 30 was sparse. And there was a drive lane right of the highway lanes. I had turned tightly, avoiding the rush of oncoming cars, and straightway began to accelerate. It seemed to me that I had length enough to match the speed of an eighteen-wheeler creeping up on my left behind me—time to match his speed and then to pass him just before merging into his lane ahead of him.

When I thought I'd both paced the truck and pulled ahead,

I eased left. The timing was perfect; in less than two seconds the drive lane ended.

Suddenly a horrible grinding shook the Ridgeline. I bore right, humped over gravel and weeds and a narrow ditch, and came to a full stop. The engine kicked and died, while that eighteen-wheeler also hit his brakes too and, amazingly, stopped no more than his own length ahead of me.

I got out. We both did. We stood, then, looking at the damage done to my much smaller truck. Ah, me! Metal was gashed, torn and twisted all the way from my back door through the panel that covered the side of the bed. My left rear tire had been not merely punctured; it was ravaged, ripped to shreds. The trucker's wheel lugs—which projected some five inches beyond the fender of the wheel well, beyond the body of his cab and the front bumper too—had chewed my red Ridgeline as the giant once meant to chew Jack's rib cage and his intestines, dead. And look: not even a blemish on the behemoth parked in front of me, unless you count the pieces of Ridgeline blood on the lug-nuts.

A siren sounded. The cop, driving westward, had actually seen the accident from the other side of the highway.

My spirits, already tense, now sank completely into my bowels. I wanted strongly to quit this place. My bladder was suddenly full to bursting.

Well. Only several weeks earlier I changed lanes, cutting in front of a 1991 Malibu. My left rear bumper nudged his right front headlight. He called the police on his cell phone. While waiting for an officer, we chatted. He showed me several horrendous wounds which, he said, he'd gotten in a street fight in Chicago. He told me he had a fistula in his lower bowel which surgery hadn't closed. All seemed friendly enough.

"Look," he said, and popped down his upper teeth, all of them false. The man was in his early thirties, living with his parents. Troubled and helpless the man I struck: Ah, Lord, what is this? What's going wrong with me?

As soon as we were given assurances that my tumors were indeed malignant, Thanne and I made a promise together to remain close no matter what, never to hide our feelings from one another, nor ever to lie.

But now in these latter weeks I'm scared that she's feeling anger at me for all my failures. Inabilities to perform common tasks. Dramatic accidents. *Expensive* accidents.

But she isn't telling me so.

Neither cop issued me a ticket. That's okay. But Thanne has informed me that our insurance will increase more than a thousand dollars. Or else the insurance company will drop us altogether. And the cost of all my treatments is already staggering. Yes, but the university's health benefits are covering that. Why would she put those two sorts of bills together?

So, already that day I went to the agency which intermediates between us and the company (companies?) that underwrite us.

I don't know. Vanessa, the agent who was taking my statement, asked me simple, basic questions—the same questions she'd asked two, three weeks ago. She was only confirming that information, dispassionately. Nevertheless, I took things personally:

Why are people picking on me? I thought. *I'm the one who's suffering. I'm the one under terrible distress. They get to be normal. "Normal" casts me out as the stranger.*

Then, standing in that public place, divided by a low counter from a number of secretarial assistants, I burst into tears.

I couldn't help it.

Snuffling, sobbing, I murmured, "It's not my fault! This isn't my fault. I have cancer! Cancer has reduced me."

Letter #7

May 3, 2006

Dear Steadfast, Kindly Friends:

That word acquires for me an ever-deepening meaning these days. This word: "Friends."

I preached on Easter two and a half weeks ago. The Chapel of the Resurrection held something between six and seven hundred people, whom I faced as I face the sea. I concluded the sermon by making reference to the childlike, Christ-clinging attitude which lately has overtaken me. In the silence following my last word, my right hand raised to signal the strength of my trust, I stuck my left thumb into my mouth and sucked.

Then, still in that silence, I turned to my seat again, and an ocean of comfort rushed in to lift me up. For the people crowding the Chapel behind me, all those aware of my presence and willing to join me down the Jesus-road—these enveloped me, a vast congregation around my soul. And at the same time they represented you, the Dear Friends who choose to read these letters. And you represent the Jesus in whose robes I ride—and I am not abandoned.

"Friends": a communion of spirits—and of the Spirit—surrounding me like the sea, together with my most enduring paraclete, my Ruthanne, hugging hugely my body and my spirit. You darlings of my heart! You are to me a gentle, urging current: "O thou dark and deep blue ocean, roll."

Well, and even the members of my extended family (whose relationships began long ago, will-they, nil-they) grow steadily dearer and closer in the manner of a chosen friendship. This relationship has become something more than blood, something like the heat *in* the blood.

Peace to you all, and thanksgiving too.

I'm in my chemo-chair again. For the last time, I hope. After this my Tuesdays will become my own again—and in approximately two-and-a-half months we'll take pictures of my interior person, CT scans, PET scans. Then—and only then, according to my oncologists—will we come to know the effects of these treatments. We discovered the cancer a little over four months ago. It will be, then, a half year—long, long to swim these uncertain swells—before we can know the true direction of my swimming. Shoals or shores.

DAILY I WALK TO AND from my writing studio. I can measure my exhaustion by that stretch through two fields and several breaks of trees, down long, gently descending hills and then, of course, up short, steep hills. Yesterday I was forced twice to stop and bend down, hands on my knees, struggling for breath during each one of these passages. I've had a persistent, rumbling bronchitis for the last six weeks. Green sputum. This afternoon I will initiate a third sort of antibiotic. My back has become hypertender, even to the lightest touch of a hand; and my chest feels both hollow and lumpish at once. Perhaps these symptoms are as much due to the cough as to the cancer. My deep weariness must be due to the treatments (for so the physicians prophesied). Usually it's about six p.m. I hit a wall and must lie down. And there are some nights of constant wakefulness; and there are some when I am a marathon sleeper, even up to twelve hours.

I stop in my walk. The Easter season produces a scent so sensuous I want to weep. It breaks forth in whole dimensions of wild color. Apple trees are in bloom, their delicate aroma companionable, white petals like a fallen snow below the grass blades. In the spring all our wild apple trees declare themselves in their bridal dress: I count more than a score of them while standing and woofing for breath. Wild black-cherry blossoms carry a sharper, more demanding scent. The field is cluttered with every variety of jonquil (yellow) and daffodils, and the blood-red tulips: small cups and the spiking, crown-round cups. It's a feast, and I am full. I could walk again. I don't want to. The redbud trees are dawn clouds floating just above the ground. Russian olive bushes are as ravishing as honeysuckle, soon to load the air so heavily the smell seems a liquid thing. Pear trees are losing flower. Black walnuts are just this minute producing small packets of dusty leaves wound tight at the ends of their branches. And on the branches of the white pines stand clusters of inch-long, white-green candles, all of them pointing straight toward heaven to which they will shoot as fresh stems proud with new needles. By this method the tall pine grow yet a foot taller. Since moving here in 1991 I've planted an average of fifty trees a spring.

But not this spring.

Lilacs add their reliable, work-a-day, well-clothed, Victorian scent to the medley.

Wild strawberries are opening secretive, five-petaled flowers among the green shoots of fresh grass. Four-petaled the dogwood too. From the breathing mouth of Christ blows the wind that makes the fields bow down and fills my lungs with a sacred air. I move on.

I enter the last field before home. Thanne and I call this one the "Kindergarten," because this is where we've planted a single tree for each of our grandchildren. Seven trees, now. When the *kinder* come to visit I hook a large wagon behind my tractor and drive them from tree to tree, crying out the name of each as we pass it by.

"Noah, look! Your red maple!" Oldest tree in the garden, first born, first planted.

"Cassindra!" Her willow flourishes more than the others, making a graceful, long green hair.

"Emma, your fir," so bedeviled by the deer that it causes me to worry regarding the interpretation of the tree's broken progress. *No. Why should I believe in omens? She'll live a healthy, unbroken life after all. Won't she?*

I rejoice in the trees. I can be troubled by the signs. "Making Certain It Goes On," after I am no longer here to nourish them.

If I could be sure that the land would remain in the family unto the third and fourth generation, I'd ask to have my ashes sprinkled at the roots of each living tree, to become a sweet slurry of moisture, to be a cool drink for the flaming Noah-tree, honor and admiration for the thirsty Cassindra, chocolate for Emma, an eternal fruit salad for Maxwell, unfrowning peace for Anna, wise restraint for the determined Thea, knowledge for my Theron, whose knowledge of this particular Papa is both easy and incomplete.

There's a story behind all this and a fine motivation for me.

In the region of the Mississippi Delta, and in the time of slavery, the older black women would help the younger women bear their babies in the privacy of certain hidden groves. While the daughter was in labor, they brought her among the trees and washed her in a tub of water. Stroked her exploding womb. Drew her legs up into bent positions. There, in the grove and in the tub, she delivered her infant child. At the roots of a sapling tree they buried the placenta. The bloody tub-water was saved to water the little tree for the next weeks. And they gave the tree the name of the infant born.

For the brave women knew that a beloved child could be sold

away from them and its family. Therefore they loved both the offspring and the symbol-tree until the wretched loss. Ever thereafter, as long as they lived, the black grandmothers, great aunts, wise women continued to lavish affection on the living thing the lad or lass had left behind, since love must needs have a place to go and a duty to do. At the same time the children, wherever they had fetched up, could comfort themselves that love still lived on their behalf. In the trees. Their namesakes. And in spirit for their spirits.

It was a difficult comfort in a cruel and difficult world. But a comfort after all, for it was, and it is, a promise well kept.

THE HEAVENS DECLARE THE GLORY of God. Psalm 19 …

That is, like scribes the skies make an account of God's glory, whether humans can read it or not.

The firmament proclaims his handiwork. Or, better, tells stories of the actions of the Creator who created it.

Can we hear it? Well, *There is no speech, nor are there words; their voice is not heard.* So it mostly is between us and the God whom creation reveals. Nevertheless, *their voice goes out through all the earth, and their words to the end of the world.*

And now the eye of the eagle, that sun rimmed in yellow, in whose seeing I can see that the law of the Lord is perfect, reviving my soul:

For in the heavens he has set a tent for the sun, who comes out like a bridegroom from his wedding canopy, and like a strong man runs his course with joy.

His rising is from the end of the heavens, and his circuit to the end of them; and nothing (nothing!) *is hid from his heat.*

So the natural world offers mercy to those who will receive it. Wild apple trees, jonquils, tulips, strawberries.

The flaming maple tree.

Let the words of my mouth and the meditations of my heart be acceptable to you, O Lord, my rock and my redeemer.

God bless you all, friends to my Thanne and to her

laggardly

Walt

Letter #8

May 7, 2006

Friends:

I contain pain.

From the beginning I've anticipated this turn in the adventure; and, in fact, have called my Cancer Trip an "adventure" precisely because much of the experience would be (has been) altogether new to me. I have nothing to compare it to. Each fresh turn *becomes* the standard by which to understand or to measure the rest of my life.

So, too, with this pain ...

I will be busy about some common thing when pain shocks me so suddenly I snap up and grit my teeth and bark, "My God!"

I doubt it's a prayer. And yet, with no thought of my own,

truly, some inner voice immediately extends those two words into a hymn: My God! My ...

> ... *God, my Father, make me strong,*
> *When tasks of life seem hard and long*
> *To greet them with this triumph song,*
> > *Thy will be done.*

Soon I am singing it out loud, through my teeth—and only then realize how absolutely appropriate my (blasphemous?) explosion has become.

I contain pain.

Let me describe things to you as I have in the past, in the sequence of the experience.

Last week at about two a.m. Wednesday morning, I woke in a bright sweat, trembling with cold. My body was a stiff sack of pain: the big leg bones, the smaller finger joints, the cords in my neck, my taut muscles—all ruined as by the galloping hooves of horses. I lay still, dreading any motion. In an effort to ignore things—and maybe to fall back asleep—I put my earphones on and listened through several CDs of a long novel. But by three-thirty it was clear that sleep had been whupped to wakefulness. I crouched and sweat until about five a.m. Finished that novel. And finally got up to soak in a hot bath, which did, after all, make me warm again.

Come Wednesday morning: I presided and preached at a seven a.m. worship service for the Deaconess community on our campus. Thanne drove me there. Thanne cautioned me not to hug folks, nor even to shake hands with them, lest I catch some sickness they could handle easily, but which would drive me back to bed again. Thanne drove me home again.

I sat at my computer and bent to my regular labor: writing. But as the day wore on, the deep, subterranean achings returned. It grew into an interior battering hard enough sometimes to take my breath away. And so it has continued now for five days. Pain jumps from the soles of my feet into the ankles. In either place it cripples my walking. I can't describe it as sharp. Nor as a burning pain. Nor rashlike nor stinging nor biting nor cutting. Nothing caustic. Not nausea.

A whacking on the anklebone! And that particular pain lingers, tissues bruised. No rubbing eases the ache. Rubbing excites it the more. It is a team of plow horses galloping up my spine, dancing on my ribcage. Something like that. A thundering down the femur and hard against my kneecap. Or across my back, as if *I* were the horse, saddled with a crop-whip pain. This particular assault causes a whizzing at the roots of my hair. It crawls down into the lower back — burrowing wormlike into my sacrum — as a kind of sweetish squirming, so that I want to hit that bone! Hit it, rough it up, beat it back into the aching that I've come at least to comprehend.

In my skull. Behind my eyes. In my chest. And always, always, morning to night, in the dead center of my chest.

VICODIN HELPS. I AM SINCERELY grateful that my adventure waited until there were therapies and drugs to serve this sort of thing.

And we can try to dominate the pain by imagining what has triggered it. Last Tuesday afternoon I received my last chemo treatment. That dosage was greater than any ever I've received before. Could be that which has tenderized my flesh. And again, as so often before, there are shots to increase production of white cells. Bones ache at that urging of their marrows.

This is what I've been thinking: *I contain pain.* It means several things.

The first point: it's all within me. Contained inside of me. There are no external symptoms. (Except for its affect on my ambulation. I am mightily slowed down.) If I wish to discuss it (as here) people have to take my word for it. And even then I'm not sure I can communicate its quality, its intensity, its free motion through my skeleton and musculature. (Hence the exercise through several paragraphs above.)

Now, I would have thought that such enclosedness of pain would make me the Lonely Hurter. Bearing the burden all lonesomely, you see. (Well, so it was at the beginning of my diagnosis, when people scarcely knew how to react.) It should, I thought, grant me a sort of Byronic romanticism: "For I am as a weed, / Flung from the rock, on Ocean's foam to sail / Where'er the surge may sweep, the tempest's breath prevail" — poor, forsaken, solitary poet! I, in my vale of pain, enduring the greatest limitation imposed upon sentient and singular lives — this, that each must die alone.

Ah, what ineffable tragedy, to suffer alone. Unaccompanied!

Yet, no matter how often in the past I've permitted myself

to sink into such a delicious self-pity, none of this has been my response to this pain. I'm surprised at myself.

For this is the second point: I find myself consumed by a truly interesting question. Why doesn't the pain which I am forced to contain—yes, essentially alone—increase my reclusive gloom, my characteristic tendencies to melancholy? What allows me, rather, to respond with a measuring scrutiny, with a certain impersonal dissociation from this world of hurt inside my body—and with spiritual comfort after all?

Groaning helps. I recommend it. Seriously.

Transforming the pain into complete sentences, ordering it according to linguistic principles uttered aloud—especially when someone is there to listen, however little her comprehension, and especially *while* the pain is active—that helps. I am fortunate. Thanne is patient, nor does she think I'm begging sympathy.

I believe this: speak a thing, and that thing is forced to conform to the speaker's structures, language, grammar, *weltanschauung.* Authority. Even from primeval times, to know the name of something is to command it.

On the other hand, altruism is *not* my consolation. I do not draw comfort or strength from supposing that my pain serves anyone else, or else some cause beyond myself. This is not a sacrifice. It cannot come close to deeds in the imitation of Christ. (I have lived in the hope of such sacrifice and such *imitatio Christi.* This just doesn't happen to be that or to explain my genuine freedom from pain while I am *in* pain.)

The third point: perhaps the journey itself has brought

me—my soul and my quieter contemplations—to matters less selfish and more eternal. Matters in themselves larger than pain, larger than my self, yet capable of inviting me into their elevated community: a lifting of self out of self.

Death is one such "matter." A *matter*, not a being! Death (does one need to say this?) is not a living thing. It can be perceived as ungodly, since it was never God's desire that anyone should die. Evil may be a being, the Tempter a being. But death's not the enemy. (Jesus: "Those who would save their lives will lose them; those who lose their lives for my sake or for the Gospel's will find them—" Here is an *invitation* to die, albeit a spiritual death. This dying is not an enemy.) Again, death is not a being; it exists only *gegend-über* (over-against) life. Death marks the edges of life; embounderies life at its length and its breadth; it defines a life, emblazons the full shape of a life. When death can no longer be denied, but must be confronted (whether on account of a metastatic cancer or on account of a genuine encounter with the Deity) then the elemental thing itself is likewise confronted: Life! This life, bounded by death. And that might be enough for me.

But there is more.

A fourth point: finding myself, like the "world-rim-walker," at the sheer edges of life, where light and darkness contour one another, able personally to peer into the endless everlasting, I find myself as well somewhat removed from the daily pain. It is rendered less than my present conversations. See? Larger matters gathering me in; larger matters becoming common matters in my discourse—they diminish such well-defined and self-exclusive things like pain. How can something contained within my body match the death that grants life stature? Yes: this would be enough to separate me from the power of pain.

But there is more. A fifth point.

To consider earnestly a life (finally!) *un*defined by death, a life defined by nothing except Life alone (there's the puzzle that will knock pain into a purple loop, could you but give it half your mind) changes all our values, all relationships. It simplifies the self and time and purposes.

I have been a Christian for most of my life. My experiences in the faith have granted me various kinds of communion with the Christ. But this present experience introduces me (not merely my mind, but my whole person) to the Life that defines life, and defines, therewithal, my own life. Defines my *now*, and all my being hereafter.

Who, existing in such an arena, light within light surrounded by the First Light, could feel overpowered by a physical pain which is contained in—reduced to—a six-foot, one-inch standing dust, Walt Wangerin, Jr.? Nevertheless, the defining of Christ glorifies neither me nor my life. It glorifies him *as* Life. I am made most small. A likely and consoling size to be. I am set free of the burdens of size and glory and heroism and righteousness, all of which characterize the Life of Christ Eternal.

I contain pain.

Pitiful pain, reduced to a pitiful thirteen-stone-weight piece of clay—the matter left with the spirit has departed.

It's LATE NOW. I NEED to stop. This has begun to feel more intellectualized than experiential, though it arises from significant, continuing experience. And it's larger than I can wholly embrace. I'm finding my way, my friends — as much by writing this letter as by my more private, diffuse contemplations.

And I am grateful that you have taken the baby steps with me, even into a fourth page....

Walt

Letter #9

May 23, 2006

O Wonderful Company of Bright Companions —
  Peace to you and enduring health:

After her breasts had been removed, my sister-in-law told me how surprised she was that her chest became so chilly. A double mastectomy had taken away those twin cushions which had been, she hadn't realized, such efficient insulations. A person is seldom aware of the double and triple duties a body part might play while still attached.

And so now it is with me, though most of my external flesh is intact. That final chemical infusion must have packed a wicked wallop. I've lost my hair. Almost all my hair. There is the fringe of a white moustache above my lip. Odd that this should remain.

Otherwise eyelashes, eyebrows, the wires on the tops of my toes, armpits, nose-hairs, the emerging bushes in an old man's ears all gone, rendering me as naked as a baby rat. Suddenly the balmy spring — even the weather indoors — surprises me with new sensations. Summer breezes teach me the shape of my scalp. Chills carve the skullbone. Except for the skin, there's just one color left on me. Blue eyes. I'm returning to that hairless infancy when babies seem all to look alike.

Dr. Christoffer Grundmann (my colleague here, the other one besides myself who occupies a University Chair) reminds me that the monk's tonsure was meant to have the same leveling effect: no hair, no individuality; no "do," no pride. Like the branches on the Jesus-vine, none is distinguishable from the others. Well, but in these latter days a shaved scalp can *be* a "do," I suppose. Folks notice you. But what a curious fashion statement for an elderly university professor.

At their graduation, several of my students shaved their heads bald in sympathy with me: women as well as men!

BUT THAT BIT OF NEWS is the least of my purposes here. More important is to ease you regarding the pain I described in my previous letter. No, it's not gone. But now and again I'm granted a day's relief. It returns again. It can still open my nose when it strikes. But between these blithering bites of the serpent I'm able to work my garden: tomatoes, green peppers, acorn squash, broccoli, strawberries. Strawberries. Tomorrow, cancer-willing, lettuces and spinach, radishes, bush beans, beets, pumpkins,

zucchini. My garden feeds the two of us all the way into spring
next year.

Or so it has done every year in the past. I'm not sure whether
the both of us … Ach, I'll save that for another time.

There is, I'm finding, a problem with the *loss* of pain: one loses
too the blessing of a primary, all-consuming focus, and that loss
has several unhappy consequences.

Serious pain relieves me of responsibilities. How can I work
when I can scarcely even name the task? — let alone unravel its
complexities? And no one else would expect work from one dou-
bled up in pain. I am by nature (and by a lifelong guilt) a driven
man. I get anxious doing nothing. I can't help it. Like the spring
that breaks its restraints, I jump up, start to pace, scribble notes,
make time out of no time, and strive to make my use of time worthy of that time. Pain overcomes guilt! And great pain forestalls
even the fear of blame. Losing it, I lose a certain consolation. Do
you see?

The first consequence of the desertion of pain is negligible:
lesser succor for smaller personal faults. An internal itch. This
affects no one but myself.

The second, however, requires confession because it affects
other people, especially those who live the suffering with me.

I am patient in pain. I can lie still and watch old television
without the need to comprehend it. The flickering light is enough,
the noise — the global positioning which the single source of light
and sound afford me: *it is right there; therefore I am right here.* I doze and

groan. Nothing troubles me except the one big thing. How can I complain about a lack of salt when I lack an appetite? Or get irritated by a certain tone of voice I might have thought sarcastic when all tones sound the same to me? Or criticize someone else's slowth when my own life has almost stopped?

Now, then: remove that "one big thing" and what's left? You'd like to think that one's conversations with death under the pressure of a felonious pain should elevate a person's spirit when he ascends into sunlight again, right?—purify it, you know, as in a refining fire. Wellllll, at least in my case righteousness isn't given as a reward for mere endurance. Still and still, at my returning to myself, I gotta work at righteousness. For out from under the cancer-rock crawls the same-ol' same-ol' ... Walter.

Confession: I'm returning to my pickier self, grumpier, fussier, graceless, ungrateful. Hypercritical. Deaf to human nuance, presuming insults no one meant, and, no longer patient in pain, consumed by my precious, superior, artistic labors.

Awareness is a good first step. Confession, the second step. And forgiveness (surely!) follows as the third—and right here is the sequence that can genuinely change a fellow. At his core. It may be fully as difficult to endure the pain, however great. It is certainly more effective. But (this is the twist and the gist, I think, of what I'm getting at) often it takes the pain—and then its cessation—to recognize one's need for what was always available but what had always seemed of small significance before. Surely, surely, high drama and the extremities of human experience are the real catalysts for change, right? So says conventional wisdom.

TV and movie plots. A host of personal "witnesses" in church. The automatic question of news reporters, the anticipated and automatic answer: "I'll never be the same again."

Well, I can only speak for myself. What first enters the drama also exits the drama. Who goes in comes out, one and the same.

Not the drama, but this ought to effect a genuine change in me: to know myself (how*ever* the knowing's acquired); bravely to confront the truth of self (*gnothe sauton* the Greeks demanded: "know thyself"); to repent my iniquitous truths face-to-face with Truth Himself; by whom to be as radically transformed as one who has been raised from the dead.

Now *that* drama, gentlefriends, is altogether too private to make the morning news.

Walt

P.S. Several of my children laugh at my various antics when they were children: that while they sat at breakfast I danced in the kitchen and in my underwear. That I stayed outside picking plums in a plum tree during a thunderstorm so violent that Thanne had commanded all four children into the basement for their safety. That several of them would rather ride with me at the wheel than with their mother. "Your driving was exciting!" My driving was headlong and peppered with a grim, explosive, delightful language, ha, ha, ha!

I don't mind these silly taunts. My kids love me.

But it is their memory of one particular father-habit

which fills me with a humble gratitude every time I hear it. This one I can't chalk up to goodness, but to Godness dwelling in me.

Often (so they tell it) after I had disciplined a child of mine — by raking her with angry eyes ("little beady eyes," Talitha called them), by shouting out her idiocy, sometimes by spanking the more egregious sins — often, I say, I would show up in their bedrooms at the end of the day. I'd walk in without turning on the lights and ask whether the punished one was still awake. "Yeah, Dad." Then, softly, I would apologize for my behavior that day.

I too recall these repeated confessions. In my memory I am a haggard creature, tentative, dreading the loss of my daughter's love. How could I be such a stentorian boomer? Why did I always lose control?

Daughter Mary, however, remembers my gesture as so regular a thing that she got used to it. It became for her a pattern of persistent return — something she could anticipate even during a punishment. Punishment, then, never did, nor ever could, break our family into bits.

Today Mary's three children wonder why she always comes into their nighttime bedrooms to tell them that she loves them.

"I get it from you, Dad."

So all along I have been confessing sins whereby I hurt other people.

And here is the sacred evidence that I have been forgiven:

those whom I have hurt by God are healed. Their wounds are closed. Not a scar remains. This I consider a miracle of the healing Christ—both grace and his face shining through the kind, continuing love of friends and colleagues and little children.

W. W.

Letter #10

June 15, 2006

Friends and Siblings and Relatives:

Thursday morning. I'm in my writing studio; Thanne's at her desk in the house. About our separate tasks, yet both of us are waiting for a telephone call which ought to come sometime this morning. Just as she has accompanied me to every doctor's appointment, we'll hear the news together.

One of my oncological doctors promised to make this call when, two days ago, I had a face-to-face consultation with him. He had meant to discuss the results of a CT scan performed a week before that consult. But then, when the three of us had sat in his examination room, he confessed that he was unable to offer us *any* specifics regarding the success or failure of the long series of radiological therapies. Hence the telephone call for which Thanne and I are now waiting—with some anxiety.

Throughout these latter weeks I have grown shorter and shorter of breath. As long as the radiation continued day by day, I was strong enough to walk from the university to the clinic, nothing abated. But now I can't climb a single flight of stairs without bending over, grabbing my knees, dropping my head and breathing, puffing, pumping and sucking fresh air into my lungs as if I'd just run up twenty flights, me and my briefcase and a stone on my back. There is no floor to my breathing. Oddly, there *is* a ceiling. I mean that when I try to inhale deeply, the upper portions of my lungs refuse to open and accept the air—and the tender ceiling against which my efforts hit does itself become irritated, chafed; so I am forced to cough. Every morning there's a whole lot of ratchet coughing. I strive to suck in a good lungful of air in order to blast the irritant out. But consider what sort of a mewling, pitiful huff is created when the irritant is not a something in one's lungs, but IS one's lungs.

Dead center, my chest is kicked with every cough.

These days I put my hand to old, familiar labor. But the old, familiar labor puts its hand to me as if I've never done it before. For example, three hours ago I attached the mower deck—a six-foot Bush Hog—behind my John Deere 5000 tractor. I do this four and five times through a summer's season. The deck comes off every time I need the tractor for plowing, hauling, using the front loader.... It goes on again whenever the fields need mowing. This pattern of the task exists in my hands, which scarcely require a brain. They do, however, require lungs. Early this morning, having to pause to breathe, pausing over and over (as we say) to "catch my breath," lengthened the simple job to one of heavy labor lasting not fifteen minutes, but more than an hour. And, of course, there is no hair to soak up my sweat: my lashless eyes sting; my bald head rains sweat down my face and jaws and neck and throat; my unshaven (but hairless) armpits put forth an altogether ribald odor.

On Tuesday, then, one of the chief questions we brought to the doctor was: "What's happening to my lungs, that now, months after my last radiological treatment, I'm losing my breath so easily and catching it with such difficulty?"

He couldn't say.

Back in March, after the last treatment, he had discussed "Time" with us. He told us that the good effects of the radiation would continue working inside my lungs for weeks, if not months. "It needs Time, you see, to finish its work." This is why we didn't take a look inside my mortal body until about two and a half months had passed. And therefore "I can't tell you if the treatments were working at all until—"

—until two days ago, June 13, last Tuesday.

BACK IN MARCH, HEARING HIS admonition to "be patient," I had responded with a sigh. "Oh, but it is hard to wait so long, not knowing."

I think the doctor thought that I was asking all over again

why we had to wait so long. He began all over again to explain the necessary medical reasons....

I interrupted him. I said, "I know. I know. I'm only just saying that it's hard to wait so long in ignorance."

For the third time he launched into the same explanations. It made me weary. What? Were we miscommunicating? Was I a dunderhead?

"No!" I said. "I'm talking about Time too," I said. "It's just, I'm only making an observation, is all."

I peered into his eyes. I held his silently for a moment. "Just this, Doctor. I need only to *say* this. To say and to be heard: that it is hard to wait, not knowing."

The good man. He paused. Neither did he remove his eyes from mine. Finally he said, "I'm sorry."

I nodded. It was enough—

—UNTIL LAST TUESDAY, WHEN he confessed that he didn't yet have the information, and so couldn't tell us what was shutting down the fullness of my breathing.

This is how that meeting went: our doctor came into the examining room, shook hands with each of us, sat, opened my file, read it. Read it to himself, producing a whistle-breath through the hairs in his nose. Then he flipped back and forth among the pages. Then he turned, paused, and began to talk. He had a written report of someone *else's* reading of the scan; but they had not sent the actual pictures over. What about the tumors, I wondered; but my ability to frame questions was muddled by anxiety. His comments suggested to me that the tumor in my upper breast was not gone.

When Thanne asked whether it was much diminished, he said that he would have to look at the pictures himself.

When would that be?

He said he could look at them on Wednesday, yesterday. That he also wished to consult with my two other doctors, the Chemical One and our own family physician. That he would telephone us on Thursday morning with the news.

But while we were still there, he offered us a noncancer reason for the shortness of breath. Might be a temporary tightening in the lungs, in which case it would pass as Time went on.

A pretty big batch of news, one is waiting on, you see.

Here's my guess regarding this stuttering approach to information. Tumors remain, even if they have shrunk a measurable amount.

I'm guessing too that this is a problem more serious than the doctor wanted to communicate two days ago. Not till he could take out a pencil and point directly to certain shadows on the CT pictures. *There. You see? It is beyond my personal capacities.* And maybe the tumors—and their neighborhoods—have now received the full extent of radiation that the tissue can abide; so we can't go back to this same method. What options would be left? Well, that remains vague. Good reason to consult with other doctors first.

All this is guesswork, of course. But all this is just what we do, isn't it? I'm still talking about Time. When there is too much of it. When the thing that hangs in the balance is as significant as one's life. When Time drives itself between our desire to know and our actual knowing: we build possibilities upon the slimmest evidence, build according to our characteristic tendencies (euphoric, melancholic), working toward a sort of hollow knowledge —

Well. So, okay.

And okay! The phone's ringing.

THANNE AND I PICKED UP at the same time. Listened on our separate receivers. The call didn't last more than a few minutes.

It wasn't the doctor, but his secretary. She said that something has come up, which has made it impossible for the doctor to be in his office today. He can't speak to us today. He'll call ... tomorrow. Tomorrow. Crap.

But I need to know how to schedule my coming months!

What shall I write? I mean, what writing projects shall I commit myself to while I still have strength to write? Or can I trust in a continuing strength? — so that I can plan on several books? It makes a difference, choosing between what I want to do and what I need to do. Some things *must* be written before I die. And throughout the past winter/spring I developed the first draft of a long work which I'm calling in sadness *Akeldama*. If I'm running out of Time, then I'll need to attend to its revision. But if I shall have Time, Time, I can turn to a book which it would please me to spend easy Time on. A young adult novel. Fun. Give me Time and you give me still an opportunity for fun.

On the other hand, give me KNOWLEDGE and you give me the opportunity to make right decisions. And this is what wisdom is: the ability to make right decisions on one's own.

There! That's a worthy theme for this particular letter. Which I send not only to the friends whom I have addressed throughout this adventure, but also to physicians who choose to know more than they allow a patient to know. What right have you to choose *for* me? Keep KNOWLEDGE from me and you keep from me several things equally as important: FREEDOM and WISDOM and CHOICE.

Doctors, please! Pay attention to this. Your "wise" silence restricts my dignity, my own wisdom; it delimits the fullness of my humanity. These are no small things you choose to remove from me, almost as if you chose surgically to cut out some necessary organ.

Enough said.

Walt

Letter #11

A Letter Never Sent

THANNE PRAYS FOR ME. SHE prays God for my healing. Nor does she mince her words, my brave paraclete. She does not approach the Almighty sidling slantwise, but head-on, fearlessly, fully aware of the elemental difference between her and her Creator. He who made her and has the power to blink her out of existence. No matter.

"Please, Jesus, heal Wally."

Not so much as an "If it is your will, O Lord."

She wants this healing to *be* his will, and so she prays.

Yet her manner is not fierce. Nor is it demanding or angry or desperate or wheedling. It has all the shining trust of a child. And I don't blame her supplications.

But I find it almost impossible to join her. I cannot pray for myself. I do not pray for my own healing.

O Thanne:

When we sit together at Holy Communion, while other worshippers file forward to the altar and sunlight floods the sacred nave, I know what you're doing. I know the meaning of your bowed head, and your closed eyes, and the straight line your mouth takes in concentration.

There is a hymn I've come to associate with my death. It moves me when we sing it as a congregation—while you sit beside me in prayer:

> *There in God's garden*
> *stands the Tree of Wisdom,*
> *Whose leaves hold forth the*
> *healing of the nations:*
> *Tree of all knowledge,*
> *Tree of all compassion,*
> *Tree of all beauty.*
>
> *Its name is Jesus,*
> *name that says, "Our Savior!"*
> *There on its branches*
> *see the scars of suffering;*
> *see where the tendrils*
> *of our human selfhood*
> *feed on its life blood.*

And then this verse:

This is my ending,
>   *this my resurrection;*
into your hands, Lord,
>   *I commit my spirit.*
This have I searched for;
>   *now I can possess it.*
>>   *This ground is holy....*

At that verse I always begin to weep silent tears. I choke up and can only listen while others sing it. You scoot close beside me so that our bodies touch, hip to shoulder. I see tears trembling on your eyelashes. I think: *Thanne, you must sing this song at my funeral.*

All heav'n is singing,
>   *"Thanks to Christ whose passion*
offers in mercy
>   *healing, strength, and pardon.*
Peoples and nations,
>   *take it, take it freely!"*
>>   *Amen! My master!*

Even now, writing the verses out and hearing the tender music in my mind, I'm inclined to cry again. For the astonishing, seventeenth century metaphor: Christ himself is the Tree in the Garden: *Yet, look! it lives! its / grief has not destroyed it / nor fire consumed it.*

Here. This is the closest I come to a word regarding my healing:

a declaration that in the end it will surely come. But I am consoled, my dear wife, by your persistent praying.

WHY CAN'T I BRING MYSELF to pray for my own healing? Well, it seems a bit presumptuous.

Not that I don't believe in the prayer's effect. I've prayed the same prayer for others, with neither hesitation nor skepticism.

While I served my inner-city congregation, an elderly woman would sometimes arrive on a Sunday morning sooner than anyone else. She knew that I'd be there alone. She was seeking me out. Marie Lander: short, terrified of thunderstorms, given to sudden, explosive laughs, a sly cut to her eyes, a shout-singer—and periodic headaches so forceful as to strike her blind.

"Pastor. Come lay hands on me."

I set no great store by my hands. There never occurred a transformation in me. Plain Walt obeyed a dear, plain woman. Neither did I scorn her or think my actions a mere semblance. This wasn't playacting. I believed that we put ourselves in the way of the Lord.

So, in the dawn darkness of winter, I would position myself behind her, the both of us standing, her head no higher than my chest. I would place my hands, palms down, on either side of her head. The pads of my fingers felt the netting of a wig. Softly, then, I prayed for the descent of the Spirit specifically upon my friend Marie, that it might take the place of her headache.

According to her, it never failed. My ministration always healed Miz Lander.

No: I sought no psychological cause. I did not play with notions that our morning sessions might have a placebo effect. Simply: we prayed and she was healed.

Yet I cannot pray the same prayer for myself.

I know from the letters I receive daily—from individuals as well as from whole congregations—that there must be more than a thousand people beseeching heaven on my behalf. And I'm filled with gratitude for their faith and their affection. Truth be told, I hold all these supplications as lightly as I held the task Marie used to give me: it may be, it may not be—either way, who am I to require or else to determine the outcome?

Is this a certain faithlessness on my part?

Is my cool (lukewarm?) conduct in such a sea of sweet petitions a surrender to sickness and the inevitable?

Well, perhaps this is a genuine explanation: I don't fear death. I am peaceful in my present state. I feel no urgency for change. Why pray for one particular outcome when *whatever* God chooses for me is altogether fine by me?

Our children have grown into their adulthoods. They've surpassed the age at which I had considered myself reasonably clear concerning my paths in life. They've brought beautiful grandchildren here to us.

People may grieve my absence. This whole affair is so much harder on Thanne than it is on me. There's a good purpose for her praying—and for the extension of my life.

For myself (as you know right well, Thanne) life has seldom

been a positive proposition for me. I've lived too much in sorrow and a hypersensitive melancholy. Almost every task before me has caused such tension that I gag and nearly throw up. The fact that I do them well means nothing. The fact that I have genuinely been called to do them, that means so much more, because I have no choice in the matter: preaching, lecturing, leading meetings as a pastor, teaching anything from confirmation classes to courses here at Valparaiso. So what's to lose?

Look: Shadrach, Meshach and Abednego, just before Nebuchadnezzar threw them into the fiery furnace, made a statement of faith so magnificent that I don't think there was another such until Jesus himself lived out the same faith.

Nebuchadnezzar in furious rage commanded that Shadrach, Meshach and Abednego be brought in.

"Now, if you are ready to fall down and worship the statue that I have made, well and good. But if you do not worship, you shall immediately be thrown into a furnace of blazing fire, and who is the god that will deliver you out of my hands?"

They said, "We have no need to present a defense to you. If our God whom we serve is able to deliver us from the furnace of blazing fire and out of your hand, O king, let him deliver us. *But if not, be it known to you that we will not serve your gods and we will not worship the golden statue that you have set up*" (my italics).

Even if God gives them no sign at all, yet they will obey him!

Whichever the case, the three young men will not break faith. Whether they live or whether they die, it is all one with them.

Even if my God should take no extraordinary measures regarding my life, I am nevertheless at peace.

They didn't pray. Simply, they stuck to the Lord God. He would do as he pleased. God was God however he chose to act.

Likewise Jesus: even hanging on the cross, dying, suffering what seemed (what *was?*) the abandonment of his Father, yet he obeyed — even unto death.

Why, resting my soul upon the everlasting bosom of my Lord, should I be any different?

Thanne, does that explain my silence on this matter? Can you receive this as faith after all, and not some shrinking doubt on my part?

This, I think, is what I do:

I live as Miz Lil lived after the death of her husband, Douglas.

"He never learned to drive a car, you know," she told me several months after we had buried the good man whose stature was no taller than hers. She was rubbing and rubbing her stomach. Caressing her womb, as it seemed to me. "He walked. He always wanted to walk. Well, and he loved to talk, is the reason. He would talk to anyone he met, dollar-proud or penniless. I hated to send him for something I needed right now, because it didn't matter how much I hurried or harried him, Douglas would always take time to stop and talk to people. Oh, Pastor. Oh, Pastor."

We were sitting in her living room, in the darkening twilight. The dim lines of her face, the rising lids beneath her eyes seemed to float her vision upward. But her conversation was a powerful agent for remembering, and I saw Douglas myself.

Miz Lil was rocking and riding the darkness. I heard the cricking of her chair.

"But he always came home. Late, untroubled, he always walked into the house again. He hung his hat with me. I never disputed his habits, no. Seems we never had cause to argue. Seems we just got along.

"So, 'Lil,' he said to me one evening. 'Where is that pie you baked for supper?'

"I said, 'In the kitchen.'

"He said, 'I think I'll have some more of that pie.'"

Miz Lil paused her rocking. "What was that pie? Mm. Why can't I remember what kind of pie that was?"

I couldn't help her. I kept quiet.

"I was resting on the sofa, you know," she said, "just where you're sitting. We were watching the TV. I heard him go into the kitchen and open a drawer, for a fork, I suppose — then I must have dozed a little.

"I woke up suddenly. It wasn't any noise what woke me. The quiet. It was the quiet woke me. I don't know how to explain it. Such a peculiar quiet, and a stillness in my body.

"Douglas was lying on the floor. Perfectly still, you know. I saw the piece of pie on the arm of his chair, partly eaten, and the fork was there. He must've gotten up and was coming to tell me something; but the house was quiet now. I can't explain the feeling to you. Between the chair and the sofa Douglas just lay down and died."

We were in full darkness now. Miz Lil was rocking again: *crick, crick.* Her shoulder kept catching a piece of moonlight, then dropping it. *Crick, crick.* And that other softer sound, an almost inaudible whispering of fabric—ah. Rubbing her womb.

"He always come back, Douglas did, always untroubled. But he hasn't come back home this time.

"And he's left an ache like a stone in my stomach.

"Pastor, the aching—this hasn't left me, always, always there."

My hands stole to my own stomach. I recognized her stone.

"The doctor keeps telling me that he wants to operate on my heart. They always said that I had a poor heart, even before Douglas died. Well, and I do get tired these days, and I have to lie down more often than not. But I don't want no cutting."

The rocking stopped. Moonlight on her shoulder.

Then: "Pastor?"

"What?"

"Is something wrong?"

"No."

"I've gotten used to the ache by now. It's all right. It's all right. I call it a friend to me. This aching reminds me of Douglas. Mm. There is a gravestone in Oak Hill Cemetery, on his grave, you know. But it's a sort of stone in me too. The children can mourn by that stone in Oak Hill. This one is mine. The widow's stone."

Crick, crick, crick. She rides a gentle memory deeper into darkness.

"Douglas used to fish. He and his friends. He sometimes get a nice catch of cat fiddlers and bring them home. Or bluegill. Or else buffalo, we call them. Pastor?"

"Yes?"

"You're crying."

"Ah, Miz Lil."

"I cry sometimes even now. Alone. In my bed at two of a morning."

I heard the soft rustle of fabric.

Crick, crick, crick. The moon had fallen into a pool on the floor.

"But he always comes back again, Pastor. I think about that. Maybe late, but never troubled. Here. In the grief-stone, the re-membering stone. This is the place of my Douglas now. It's com-fort, you know. He hangs his hat with me."

Crick, crick.

THANNE. THIS IS WHAT I do. Like Lil, I have my tumors inside of me. I bear them as a kind of thinking place. My dying, you know. A kind of memory before the fact. Good company.

I love you.

Wally

Letter #12

My friends:

Swift on the heels of my previous letter comes this one. Forgive me the clutter. Or read whatever suits you best. Or don't. For you truly know best your time, your intentions — and the things that serve them both.

It's Saturday morning, June 17. I wrote that last letter two days ago, Thursday morning. Suddenly, being so drawn to the topic, just now curling my fingers over the keys, I feel I'm writing a book; that these letters are beginning to be chapters in a book — a very loosely associated book, of course, except for these two particular letters, which must follow one upon the other as closely as I can make them go (though Kathy Sutherland won't be here until Monday, and she's the one who has the computer and the knowledge to email this to you).

Well. But because on Thursday I wrote words of admonition to those doctors who hold information both regarding and concerning (that is, information important to) their patients; and because my words touched upon my experience with a particular doctor; and because this particular doctor *did* call after all with the information for which we had been so hotly waiting—I must now touch on such topics as kindness and trust and thanksgiving. Topics which can't wait. Or they would wilt in the waiting, losing force and virtue. And these topics, when they wither, drop no new seed in the ground of relationship.

"THE GOOD MAN," I CALLED him in that last Cancer Letter. He has proven that assessment (though I'd given it in a single, fleeting phrase). He has my thanks more, perhaps, than I can say.

Thursday, the same day I wrote in criticism, after Thanne and I had finished supper, after seven p.m. in the evening—surely after his workday was also finished—the doctor telephoned. Not an assistant. Himself. He had studied the CT pictures, had spoken directly with the radiologist whose report he'd read earlier, and had compared medical notes also with our family physician. He wanted to explain to us what he had found out. He didn't want us to wait any longer. He wanted to prescribe a new medication. Prednisone.

And fully as much as that medication might help my breathing, the doctor's kindness helped my spirit.

Doctors who practice medicine ARE medicine—especially because they invite and sustain a patient's trust. Perhaps it were enough to trust one's physician for skill, intellect, and the excellence of scientific acumen. Perhaps one considers only one's body. Perhaps one considers that this is ALL one is: a body. Well. As far as I am concerned, a serious disease invades more than the body's physical systems. For it invades by creating an entire meteorology of disturbances. (My body is much the weather around my soul!) What it disturbs, then, and tests is also all the rest of me: my character; personality; faith; morality; virtue; the spirit's gifts as well as the spirit's vacuities. I am patient. I eat what has become tasteless. I grow grumpy. I lose focus. I drive without the same alertness as before, having accidents, troubling those nearest to me. People just discovering that mine is a lung cancer ask immediately, "Do you smoke?" Or the softer version: "Did you smoke?" I am irritated by the implications. A black and silent bitterness collects in me, stinging someone: either stinging me in my spirit (because, yes, I did once smoke—but I quit in 1982, didn't I? Nearly a quarter century ago? I did, friend! I did the right thing!) Or else stinging my inquisitor by a brittle response (for in these days the one immorality that everyone can agree to criticize and deny others is smoking: SMOKING WILL KILL YOU, YOU IDIOT!) Or one can stand in despite over against folks who come with the kindest intent. "Walt!" they exclaim, "how good you look!" Before God, and in my better temper, I do not blame these blessed friends. They've associated cancer with immediate desiccations, and had anticipated finding a gaunt Walt after all. And I believe that their assessment, "How good, Walt!" is meant to cheer me, is more than mere observation. But, as I say, I stand in despite of their good assurances. For in my ears—all inside my invisible, physical storms, the heavy winds that steal my breathing—these assurances sound weak, distant, and ignorant. And this is the thorn-end of my despite: that it blames kind people from behind my false smile and my noncommittal response: "I do, don't I?"—while that black blame stings with secret thoughts: "Do you *want* me to look bad? Is this part of the play? Are you disappointed? Do you think me *less* dis-eased thereby?" No, no, no, it isn't okay to be bitter. No! Cancer does not give me freedoms others don't have. A snarking thought, even when kept internal, becomes a warm, pumping, venomous fluid that runs in one's vessels, whether bloody or lymphatic or made of the clay of the Creator—filling the vessel that one IS.

You see? My body is the weather that pervades and proves the rest of me, every spiritual part of me.

Therefore the healing of a physical disease requires remedies so much greater than scientific prescriptions, prednisone, infusions of chemicals, streams of radiation. The quality of my trust in a doctor cannot be restricted to how she/he might handle my corpus. Empirical knowledge may (or may not) change my corporeal weather to what? Back to "normal" again? But its effect upon my spirit in the meantime—the resultant defects revealed and developed in my spirit—is not changed by such scientific medicinals. How can that be healed? Better yet, what might preserve that from itself becoming dis-eased in the meantime? What more must I trust in my physician than his body-knowledge?

We are talking about kindness. We're talking about attentions to a patient's interior wrestlings.

During this entire week I've found myself surprisingly close to tears. So have I felt when Thanne and I discuss possibilities and dyings. Discussing, for example, that, as I weed my strawberry bed—and as I nip the tiny green berries from newly planted plants so that they may produce a more wonderful fruit next year—I think: *But who will eat the berries then which I cannot now? Who will come to pluck them?* Such thoughts unman me. So did I feel especially when we drove home together on Tuesday with no new news. Thanne said to me, "You should cry. You should let it out." Because I had just exclaimed, "Oh, I don't like this feeling! I hate it!" Weakness. And worse when it shows its pale face in public!

But when the doctor called on Thursday evening, and when he brought a complete report of all that he can know right now, then my urge to tears felt baptismal, my spirit's washing, warm and good—no *matter* how "good" or "bad" the news itself.

In the last letter I called him a good man. But a telephone call like his invites and sustains my trust in the man—in the *person*, do you see? As much as in the doctor. And my spirit wants, needs, aches to be a part of such an interchange. Yearns a trust more whole—more wholesome and altogether more holy—than in the physician's digits alone.

AND, BRIEFLY, THIS IS WHAT he told us:

That he has been most concerned about the major tumor beneath the mid portion of my sternum; that, according to the CT scan, it looks as if the tumor is much reduced; but that there are certain very small (he didn't say "spots") in the areas which received the radiation treatments. Now, these (could his word have been "granular"? Or "like grains of sand"?) "spots" most likely represent a condition called *pneumonitis,* a series of tiny fibril tumors caused by the radiation itself which, these tiny tumors not being malignant, do restrict my breathing significantly. Hence, the prednisone. There are two kinds of such sandy-scatterings of tumors, one transient, the other — what? In-transient? This one does not pass away with time. One lives with them. A very low percentage of radiation patients ever develop pneumonitis, he said. A tiny, distant target. Apparently, I'm an excellent shot.

But what he also said is as blessed as what I've already recounted here. And for this he has of me an even finer gratitude; for the next thing came of pure honesty. And this next bit of information was given in trust and in kindness. I mean, he could have kept it to himself until I received the more delineating PET scan, July 13.

The doctor said that there is an unlikely, but a not-impossible chance that what he views in the present, less accurate CT pictures is not pneumonitis at all, but the cancer still, malignant still, and scattered like tiny soldiers in tiny assaults on tiny parts of my northerly lungs. But to ease our fears he wanted to assure us that the far greater likelihood was pneumonitis after all.

"Eighty percent," he said. "Higher," he added. "Yes, higher than eighty percent, it's pneumonitis." Which, of course, translates into "twenty percent" for a continuing distribution of the cancer. But "lower. Yes, lower than twenty percent."

Aye, but I have ever been a man of melancholies. And, as I have already written, an excellent shot at targets both small and far away.

Walt

Letter #13

July 23, 2006

My dear, patient friends:

my darling family —

One of the advantages of an old man's losing all his hair (so thinks this old man) is that it clears his nostrils and his ear-holes of four mighty bushes. One of the disadvantages of the same fellow's hair's returning is ... Well, you get the picture.

I keep rubbing the slow stubble growing on my skull, not having had this experience since I was too young to know (or to care about) the experience. I am astonished at the darkness and the rich thickness of the new hair on the backs of my fingers, my hands and arms. I'm carpeting. Whether the new head-hair is noticeably different in texture I'll have to let you know.

Today is Sunday, July 23. During this last week Thanne and I met with both oncologists, each in his and her own examination rooms and offices and cities. I've had the PET scan scheduled a while ago, after the CT scan which I've already mentioned in these letters. Also, on Thursday I was given a series of pulmonary tests to take a definite measure of the reductions of my breathing.

The news from the PET is good. Both physicians confessed themselves happy with the effects of the therapies upon the tumors. They've shrunk decisively. They're still there. The one sitting central in my chest continues to show activity. Its metabolism has not been shut down. But the activity is much reduced. What was supposed to happen happened. Nor were there any new tumors discovered in the areas between my brain stem and my thighs.

(We had scanned the brain early. "Just to get a base," she said. "A base?"

"Against which to compare future scans. It's not improbable that this particular cancer may metastasize to the brain. Or the spinal cord.")

But both doctors were cautious in their optimism. Tiny tumors do not appear even on the PET, one told me. We've scheduled another PET, then, for three months hence.

The pulmonary tests, however, have raised a different set of problems. At my age, weight and size, I should be inhaling something over 5 liters of air with each breath I breathe and blow. But the fact is that I can inhale no more than 2.45 liters. The volume my lungs can accept is less than half of what it could before the radiation began. Pneumonitis has now become the established diagnosis. Portions of my lungs have been rendered useless by the healing/killing rays beamed into me while I lay perfectly still on a flat and narrow board, my arms tight against my thighs. Those great glass eyes peering into my innards, then cranking around my body for this angle and that, shooting through good tissue to hit the bad.

It may still be transitory, the oncologist offered in a spasm of glass-half-full benignity. He had not mentioned this particular side effect before we began the treatment. I don't know what we might have done if he had. Perhaps he thought that the chances were minimal, and why trouble the fellow about to put his lungs into the hands of technicians day after day. (Forgive the snidery.) Since these readings are not his specialty, he is sending me to another doctor altogether. A pulmonologist. New examinations. New treatments.

When I try to breathe deeply, I sense something like a rough roof in the upper tissues of my lungs. Hitting that roof excites a rush of irritations. The irritations drive me to coughing. And the level of that roof, and the consequent capacity of my lungs, both seem to have dropped in the last several weeks. I can feel the diminution. It affects my strength and endurance. My daily measurement is still the walk from the house to my writing studio: a slow, slow ambulation. (*Very* slow, if you ask Thanne, who will swiftly leave me behind—as once in my headlong intensities I used to do to her.) I stop, exhausted, every four or five strides; bow my head between my knees, feeling a racing heart; puff and puff to stuff enough oxygen into my blood that I might rise and walk again another five strides.

And fits of gasping now interrupt my normal talking. I am that, a talker. I live by words. I want to bat at these sudden suckings the way a picnicker bats at flies. But these my woofings do not fly away. I huff and cough and do not speak — while others jump into the breach, cutting off the second half of my sentence, the weightier half of the sentence, I am sure.

I WRITE LIGHTLY. FOR THE most part, my tone reveals my mood. Well, but it's when I'm not writing that other moods can overcome me.

Two days before each new oncological visit and examination, Thanne and I begin to stress. Between one visit and another we've made lists of the symptoms that wrack me. We'll ask the doctor about each one. Irregularly, but often enough, I will be laid flat with something similar to a disabling bone-and-joint flu. I've lost my appetite. Food seems such an imposition on my body. I'm losing weight (a beneficial symptom). Headaches (Thanne, do you think it *is* a tumor in my brain?). Lists like this we take with us as we drive from Valparaiso to Chesterton, where the offices of our chemical oncologists are. In hushed voices we talk:

What do you think?

I don't know. Everything.

Wally.

What?

*What will we do? What will **I** do? I can't take care of the property on my own, you know.*

Ah, Thanne, none of the children wants it.

Well.

She pauses. Then:

I have to think about selling it.

I pause. Then:

I'll miss it, Thanne. This is the first time I've ever felt home.

Miss it? Wally — you'll be dead.

I know. Well — I miss it already.

And we pray together. And I can't express how grateful I am that Thanne comes along on every one of these visits.

THE LAST SEVEN MONTHS HAVE bound Thanne and me to one another more tightly, more devoutly and sweetly than (perhaps) ever before. Topics between us have become the more elemental. And we cannot *not* be honest. But talking itself has become less necessary. And the last seven months have shown us (actually, have astonished us and have humbled us by) the wonderful community of friends who fill our house with intelligence and love and generosity and companionship and holiness, faith, prayer, humor, steadfastness. You people! — a bright and complex patchwork of individuals, never a mere slurry of colors. You have made yourselves — your selfs, your spirits, each your particular disposition and talents — well known to us. Here surrounding us; here in our kitchen as we read your emails and your snail letters together. And we receive your presence, a dear and nourishing thing. Oh, thank you for the kindness. For the revelations of your selfs, and for your love.

In other words, the experiences of the last seven months have produced a marvelous garden of enduring benefits. Good news on top of good news.

And so then, with regard to life's quality: there still are restraints and restrictions. This is to be expected, isn't it? But they cannot help but be balanced by the blessings discovered under the surgence of life in the life/death zone.

I will teach this fall. I will write. We can make plans.

SINCE MARCH I'VE BEEN REDEEMING the passage of slow time by contemplating the things I would/will do, should I survive the cancer. Like getting a dog. Like traveling less without suffering the pinches of guilt for having to decline invitations. I will not feel bad for taking time away from public commitments in order to give time to Thanne and the children and the grandchildren, to give time to my writing (an occupation which requires, after all, very little lung capacity). And maybe I'll buy a motorcycle to save gas money. (Well, that at least is my most public reason.)

But again (I have to say it again): I find myself somewhat sorrowful to lose the riveting focus which death's likelihood provides a sick old man. Now, together with all my resprouting hairs, there rushes back a sea-tide of all the little things that hector daily living —the krill that clouds and crowds the waters once the whale is gone. Perhaps that indicates another benefaction which I ought to draw from the previous seven months: stick, Wally, to the sense of the proximity of death in order to recognize (at some spiritual and perdurable level) how little *are* the little krill—even as little as dying (always, always) is near. Here.

WE DON'T TALK OF CANCER'S "cure." Surely we don't have that right, given what continues in my body. But even should all signs of it vanish, this easier condition remains a "remission" of the disease. It's a wise distinction. My sister-in-law—she of the double mastectomy, five years in remission—still bewares the specter hovering above her. This isn't morbidity. It is evidence of the weight of her surgical and recuperative experience past. It is her proper recognition of the statistical facts, that having had cancer once makes the possibility of her having cancer again very high.

There still will be things to write about in the coming months. How many people grieving a serious loss discover that the public's tolerance for the *continuance* of their grief is short and shortly unsympathetic. ("Get over it, already.") But true friendship remains through the more boring, repetitive extensions of sorrows even after the excitement of the new crisis is past. The public—when it is confronted with an unfinished grief long after it, the public, has finished with the griever—begins to avoid her as a nuisance, and to blame her as a mope too much in love with her black weeds.

No. I'm not implying that I occupy such a position, neglected by friends. Only this: a crisis drops long roots and continues to bear seed long after its first flowering. This too, the lengthening, seesawing experience: I want to observe this part of my adventure fully as I have contemplated any other part.

Thank you for prayers. Thank you, boundless congregation of faithful people, for prayers.

Love,

Walt

Letter #14

A Letter Never Sent

THAT FELLOW WHOSE 1991 MALIBU I bumped while changing lanes last May? The man with whom I shared pleasantries, my cancer against his multitudinous maladies? A body torn up by two back-alley poundings in Chicago, an incurable fistula in his bowel which kept introducing severe infections? Toothless, bound to leg braces (which is why he didn't get out of his car while I knelt at the driver's window in order to chat with him)? The thirty-year-old whose car was already a bent-metal mess, quite capable of driving away when the cop and our twenty-minute's conversation came to an end — remember him?

He's suing me.

The trial date is set for Friday, October 20, at one p.m.

I know where to go. I've been to the courthouse often enough as an innocent man — nobody attaching payment to my blame.

Ach!

Letter #15

August 8, 2006

Friends

> *and Sweet Folk*
>> *and Family*
>>> *and Familiars More Elfin:*

A LITTLE NEWS TO TELL you since last I wrote—and the confession that sometimes the good word will cause us, faster than a bad word, to overleap present information and imagine a fairer circumstance than *any* word should have justified. One should never be too soon euphoric. This news isn't what you'd call "good."

The volume of my inhalations remains what it was—about half what it ought to be. But two weeks ago my breathing took a sudden turn for the worse, carrying me quickly to a new physician, the pulmonologist recommended by the radiation oncologist (doctors piling on top of doctors). He ordered another CT scan, one of different properties than those I've been used to. These new pictures showed a sizeable blood clot in my right lung. Straight into the hospital he sent me. How long? Not long. Not much over a week. A *week*? School starts in two weeks.

In the hospital I would begin to receive hypodermics of blood thinners. There they could watch and adjust the dosage.

"Take a break," he said, knowing nothing of my guilt factor at *any* break.

I was admitted and given a bed.

In a few days I learned that if I wanted to go home, I'd need a visiting nurse to give me the shots. Not only too expensive, but it was only the hospital stay that the insurance company would cover.

In another day I asked, "But what if I gave myself the shots?"

Hum. No one had thought of that. Had I ever given myself shots before? A diabetic, maybe?

Well, no. But I could learn. It's my own body.

I stuck an orange once and learned straightaway—and now I shoot myself in the stomach several times a day. But my blood now is very thin. My tummy blooms like a rose garden of dark red and purple blossoms, a new one for every puncture.

Also, I've become that elderly man in the grocery store who wheels canisters of oxygen behind him and wears tubes up his nose, double faucets pumping a sparkling air through my sinuses down my throat, easing my heart of its thirst. I wear this thing all the time. I sleep with it.

The pulmonologist has nominated three other potential causes for this breathlessness. We will, as I understand it, eliminate them one at a time.

But it is not impossible to live at half-breath. When I can I'll begin to wean myself. Walk. Walk a step, stop a step, breathe a step. And, you know, wave my arms. Flex my hands. Exercise. That sort of thing.

And if I grow impassioned teaching, well, *then* the oxygen can charge the emotion and sustain the emoter. As always at this time of the year I do so dearly look forward to teaching — to the relationship teaching can establish with my students. This is some of my best medicine. This is motivation: not to give in to infirmities, but rather to press beyond them even for the sake of a community of excellent minds and hearts.

The pulmonologist put a small device onto one of my fingers, then took my arm and led me down one corridor and up the other. He kept reading the finger-machine. But I simply could not keep up the pace. Here is the first doctor who has spent time actually checking the breathlessness I've been fussing about so long. He is a grim beadle of a fellow, wholly impersonal, and forthright about anything in his mind. Nothing's withheld. Nothing's sugared. At the end of our trek he shook his head. What's the appropriate physiological term? I don't know. In effect he said that the oxygen exchange through my lungs into my bloodstream was critically low. Hence my new companions, silvery metal canisters, 40 inches tall, hissing like an angry cat.

"Have they told you about your cancer?" he asked just before my time was up.

"Yes," I said.

"What?"

I rattled through the technical descriptions of the disease and what its present state is right now.

He listened, breathing quickly, a man of little time or patience.

When I'd finished he said: "Good answer — if you were a doctor. Did I ask you to tell me something I already know? Now what did they tell you about your life? About your future?"

I drooped my shoulders and felt helpless.

He said: "This cancer doesn't go away. This cancer will kill you, unless something like pneumonia kills you first. Get used to it. Live your life with this in mind."

So THEN: THIS BRIEF PAGE is not about reversals, despite puffings and clottings and tummy puncturings and little riders in my chest which will ride me all the way Home. Today, Tuesday the 8th of August, the breezes have been cool, the sky lightly scudded, thin clouds spinning up like scrolls, the tomatoes ripening red, soon to become sauce.

Class preparations — each its syllabus, its semester's schedule, the series of topics before us — are complete. Two weeks in advance!

Three grandkids are arriving Thursday for the weekend. I

have a keen idea for my next novel (and with a peculiar delight have spent the length of the summer researching the project). Christ is altogether more trustworthy than the leaders of this earth are proving themselves to be. Grief and fear and a pandemic of self-serving behaviors trouble the peoples; leaders increase the fear, distort the behaviors, invert righteousness, and their destructions abound. (Will I die before the war does?) These things are true. They have been true since we hid from God — even if they do seem more extreme in these latter years.

But the promises of the Lord endure forever. He and his promises — Jesus, between the making and the keeping them — these embrace Time. They give Time its edges and its shape. And it is not wrong, on days like this one, to take one's stand as well as one's rest within such Time, the anteroom of eternity. Not in order to blind ourselves to the iniquities and the woundings around us, nor to withdraw from our service on behalf of the wounded, but simply to rejoice.

It is a good day. Gladness is available. Christ is at hand.

Walt

Part

Letter #16

September 17, 2006

Good, dear Friends:

Thanne sits beside me on the sofa. She has leaned her head back and closed her eyes. It's quarter to nine in the evening, the hour when sleep overcomes her. She's tired now. The day has been both long and demanding. The TV's on, though neither of us is watching it. Thanne's zonking and I'm writing to you. It's been a while, hasn't it? And I do, you know, bear you so much in mind these days. Not as an obligation to be fulfilled, but as a communion, friends who have freely and kindly put themselves (yourselves) in the way of my own walking.

These have become my regular existence: the swelling in my neck (a kind of gross bib tied beneath my swallow and spreading down to my clavicle bones) has necessitated an ultrasound. Weekly my blood is drawn. Still I take blood thinners for the clot in my lung ("the size of a small hand"). I bruise crimson and blue. My port is flushed. The port is a small, round donut, over which the skin grows fresh. A needle the size of pencil lead breaks through that flesh and stays there to see whether the blood flows freely through the tube tucked into the body. I still take prednisone, which is causing my large muscles to shrink. And for my recurring pain I've begun to take Vicodin. Let's see: another drug called Xanax. A cough medicine with codeine phosphate. But my cough is more powerful than codeine.

Is all this interesting? It's a compulsive topic for old folk: their physical ailments. And the sundry treatments. In fact, it reflects pride. Or one-upmanship. Like having the sleeker, more powerful motorcycle. See? My medicinals out-medicinal your medicinals.

Odd, marginally related pains: my teeth. My gums. The roots' sockets and the jaw and its joint—and these precious teeth! Root canals (can this be saved?). Extractions.

Or else, there's this: once, perhaps fifteen years ago, I mentioned an odd ache to my father, who was then in his seventies. Mine was just a passing comment. But he responded with an old man's wisdom and a complete lack of sympathy. He said, "Get used to it." These pains come. Soon enough, they stay.

It's the staying that takes the getting-used-to.

I mean: until now I've met most diseases with the assumption that I would get better. During a bicycle ride through seven Midwestern states, I broke my hip clean through. Alexandria, Minnesota. The purpose of my trip was to raise money for the radio program which I hosted — to establish personal relationship with my radio audience in order to create a fuller list of listeners and to seek bequests. Already in the ambulance I determined that I would not abandon the journey. We'd find ways to keep going. I would get better.

My boss, nowhere near me, back at headquarters, demanded I come home. He even approached my wife, telling her to persuade me to quit. She told him that I make up my own mind. And I did — in spite of the frustration it caused the boss who could not control me.

After surgery, I continued the trip on crutches.

Every winter past I've lost strength in my limbs. Every spring and summer past I've regained that strength by working on our small farm. I shed winter's excess weight, lightened the color of my hair, darkened my face in the sunlight.

Now, however, a different kind of mentality is required. I will never again be able to draw a full two-lungs' worth of air. I will ever puff at a flight of stairs. This body will nevermore be what it has been, nor can I frame my knowing it according to its ability to repair itself.

The older man's advice. The newly-old man's transition: *Get used to it.*

We're not really talking about aging itself, the plain passage of the years. We are talking about the breaking down of bodies, which begins earlier or later, depending on each person's various experiences and constitutions. We're talking about another way to live, about devising new methods for confronting old Time and physical degeneration.

In fact, it presents an irony. When we are young we strive forward, peering toward and planning for the better things to come. But we base the presumptions of our forward-peering-planning on the experiences of our past, such as getting sick and getting better every time. And no one, absolutely no one can reach into our hearts to make them wiser. (Our minds might know the facts, which are observable; but our hearts continue to live in the familiar ways.)

Now I have fetched up on the shores of those "forward" years. Here there is only a strip of beach before the sea, only a limited distance into which to peer, for which to plan. Long ago I fretted about the end of my life, that it was drawing ever nearer. *Ah, look! I'm past the half. Now there are fewer years ahead than there are behind.* And later: *two thirds of my life is gone.* I could no longer act as if my Time were endless.

One gets sick and then does not get better again. A fellow finds himself boxed in: fewer future years, fewer promises to be drawn from all those many former years.

Nevertheless, *this* thing is fresh and new, this devising methods for living the diminishing life. It can (it probably has to be) as creative a passage as any writer ever wrote. And *that* grants it the possibility of depth, gravitas and fulfillments and joy.

Well, there are those who, their lives tightening around them, act as if it were prison walls closing in, intensifying their more unhappy qualities. Whereas once they might have been able to

control their natural angers, anger becomes the strongest response — and can finally be nothing but a failing device, a lion
devouring all the remaining years.

Get used to it.

I don't have the hang of that yet. I can't abolish thoughts
about the garden I'll grow better next year than the garden I
could only piddle with this year. I tend rather toward the au-
thoritarian bark than to patience and the "listening heart" which
Solomon sought of God — things I truly, truly owe my students.

My teeth hurt! My teeth are never again going to chew as they
used to (over which I seldom concern myself). So my speech these
days will get bitten and brisk, sometimes dismissive. Ah, but as
long as I make commitments to others — to teach, to sustain, to
befriend, to love: as long as I willingly and knowingly schedule
new commitments, I have no right to self-pity.

My project, then. To get good and old. Spiritually to approach my losses with the same craft and talent and devotion
which I bring to the writing of a novel, a poem, a sermon.

I remember reading the last letter of John Keats. He wrote it
to his friend Charles Brown just ten short days before he died. He
was very sick. Tuberculosis had eaten through his bloody lungs.
Keats might have been anticipating the death soon to silence him.

In this letter the poet makes a tender farewell.

My dear Brown,

'Tis the most difficult thing in the world to me to write
a letter. My stomach continues so bad, that I feel it worse

on opening any book—yet I am much better than I was in Quarantine....

I have an habitual feeling of my real life having past, and that I am leading a posthumous existence....

If I recover, I will do all in my power to correct the mistakes made during sickness; and if I should not, all my faults will be forgiven....

I can scarcely bid you good bye even in a letter. I always made an awkward bow.

God bless you!
John Keats

Thanne's in bed. She finally noticed that she'd been dozing open-mouthed for the last twenty minutes, covered and curled on the sofa beside me. So she got up, her pupils small as black beads, and dragged herself to bed. She's sleeping. The night is growing late for me as well.

Good night, good friends. The nice thing about these letters is that you can quit reading them at any paragraph. No guilt to you, no fear in me that I might have burdened or bored you.

Walt

Letter #17

October 18, 2006

YESTERDAY, TUESDAY, WE MET WITH a new oncologist, a young man of lean stature and genuine interest. He gave full attention to our questions — working through them with us rather than halting at an admission of ignorance — or the submission of ignorance.

Oh, how welcome was his unapologetic honesty and his willingness to probe beyond our limited ability to ask questions, to know what questions we ought to ask. He lingered long over my various pains, touching, questioning, making careful notations in a personal notebook.

Thanne asked, "What should we do?"

He rested his backside against the examination table and crossed his ankles.

There were two things he advised us.

"Prepare."

This was as much as to say, Put your affairs in order. He had initiated an ancient ritual of universal and significant weight.

Perhaps his youth (could he still be an intern, himself preparing for this limited, difficult field?) emboldened him more than his older compeers, making him more alert to the patient's interior experiences? Again, his clarity steadied us. It was a focus, after all. My reaction was the same as it had been the first time my diagnosis had been assured, ten months ago. Thanne seemed characterized by a kind of angular brittleness. But I can't vouch for that. Her position has not been mine.

The second thing he advised was a new prescription, to be taken twice a day, the morning and the evening. Morphine.

That did create an evident response in Thanne. Of course it did: she feared addiction. And she knew well my addictive tendencies.

But the doctor worked to console her. "Any drug that actually reduces pain has a job to do. It's good to take, but it doesn't create addictions where it is needed."

But can't it hook him accidentally?

Doctors thought so, so they withheld it. So the sick hurt and no remedy. Physicians now know better. Taking morphine after the pain has subsided, well, that's the beginning of a problem.

Our appointment had begun at three-fifteen. By four-thirty we were at our regular drugstore, filling the prescription.

I took it with no affective change, no ethereal release from our house's reality. Simply, the pain in my chest became less and less important. I expected to sleep well.

TODAY, ANOTHER BIT OF NEWS. I ought to be relieved. I *am* relieved, but it troubles me nevertheless.

My trial was scheduled for Friday, the day after tomorrow. It has always made me nervous just to think of it. Well, several thousand dollars are at stake, and at the accident itself I confessed my fault to the young man of many afflictions, as well as to the police officer. It is written into his report. Worse, the last time I appeared before a judge, my son was on trial for petty theft. Shame then, shame now — first on both of us, now on me alone.

But the insurance company telephoned this morning. There's no need for me to keep the court date.

"Why? Has it been rescheduled?"

No. It's been cancelled altogether. There'll be no trial at all. It isn't, my caller joked, on account of the brilliance of their negotiations. It was circumstances.

"Good! Wonderful!" I wanted to tell Thanne right away. "What are the circumstances?"

The man in his Malibu, crippled, toothless, awaiting surgery to close his fistula, dosing himself with quantities of morphine greater than mine will be ...

As easily as though she were quoting a market price, the

insurance woman explained the circumstances that had cancelled the trial:

"He died," she said.

I'm not keeping score. I haven't begun to read obituaries, who has died before me, the names of friends, family, colleagues, acquaintances.

But this man's death, sooner than mine, troubles me.

And there's some shame in my soul after all.

Walt

A Fourth Meditation:
Can Give Her the Gettin'

......

AT MY REQUEST MR. COLERIDGE Churchill agreed to be the president of Grace congregation. Because he couldn't leave his work at any time during the day, I often met him in his office while the children were busy in their classrooms.

Coleridge was the principal of Delaware Elementary School, grades K through 8, students aged five through thirteen.

His wife taught at a different school. Elfrieda raised her third-grade children with a certain severity. "Our people must pull themselves up by their own bootstraps!" she said. "They cannot live on blame and handouts."

Though they both had been trained the same, and both the Churchills were educators, the manners with which they performed their jobs were starkly different.

Of her husband Elfrieda would say with some heat: "He's too liberal. He will not stiffen the spines of our children!"

Our children: this couple was African American, members of the black inner-city congregation which I served. *Our* children because she meant those whom her old-fashioned propriety still called "Negroes."

And yes. Elfrieda was right. Coleridge *was* "liberal," tender with his laughing host of pupils, but therefore beloved of them all. He went about the school with a pocketful of dimes. In his secretary's office was a large popcorn popping machine. Delaware (its principal, the truth be known) sold popcorn for 10 cents a bag. This is how he learned the names of every pupil. Which is a method, I believe, as persuasive as his wife's, who would rather turn her third-graders into diligent troops.

THE PRINCIPAL WAS TALL, MADE even taller by an explosion of greying afro yet four more inches above his head. His arms were as long as the ropes of grappling hooks. His complexion had the cast of polished walnut. Coleridge smiled. He murmured when he spoke. And his laughter came as distant thunder.

Once in early December, when the school was festooned with Christmas baubles and greenery, I entered through a door which opened into a long hallway. There, a good fifteen yards away, was Mr. Churchill, surrounded by a flock of children. He noticed me. He raised his arms to greet me. And up with his arms, attached to his arms like Christmas ornaments, rose five kids, three to one side and two to the other, who kept hanging high like happy sausages.

And Coleridge laughed. In the cavern of his chest, that rumble of thunder.

He told me of Elfrieda's history which, he said, might explain her present displeasure with her race.

She'd grown up in a family unable to support the child who wanted to attend college. Therefore, "she pulled herself up by her own bootstraps, as it were." She took herself to the institution that could train her. She talked herself through an unlikely registration. She worked all the years she studied, responsible herself for tuition and her livelihood.

What she was by nature; what she had experienced (proof of the value of her sterner stuff), she would inculcate in every child for which she was now responsible.

Well, she had the power. This woman could turn and fold her arms and spear a pastor with her eyes alone. Something like sunlight beamed from the tops of her cheeks and pierced him to his guilty heart.

Altogether too liberal, sir.

THEN, JUST BEFORE THE CHRISTMAS holidays, Coleridge asked whether I might drop by Delaware. Yes, that very day, if I could. He had something to tell me — but in private.

He met me at the front entrance, then walked me down empty hallways back to his office.

I think that the buzz of the children studying consumed the

man's attentions. He didn't speak. Our footfalls lent rhythm to that music behind the closed doors.

We turned a corner. Another hall, at the end of which was the principal's office. Coleridge slowed his motion. In fact, the tenor of his whole body changed into something watchful.

When I looked forward I saw the cause of it. In the distance sat a small white child on the floor, her back against the wall. Her head was bowed, her arms around her knees. We came very near to her. She glanced up at our coming, but immediately buried her face in her hands.

We stopped in front of her. But the principal was not looking down on her. He was keeping his gaze straight ahead, as if all his thoughts were somewhere else. We stood that way until the white child looked up again.

"Ohhh, Etta May," Coleridge said to the hallway, his murmur filled with sad compassion.

Her name! She looked down.

So porcelain white was this child that I could see the blue veins where her skin was stretched over fine, tiny knees. Her hair a melancholy cloud. Eyebrows so white as to seem to disappear.

"Oh, Etta May. She's sad. Because she wants something."

Now the child fixed her eyes high on the face of the tall man. How magical! He was right. He knew.

"But I can't give her what she wants. No, I can't."

A widening of her eyes. A quick intake of breath.

"But," said Coleridge Churchill, "I can give her the gettin'."

He reached into his pocket, then reached to shake the tiny

white hand of Etta May, and when their hands parted she had a dime.

"What needs telling," he said to me after we'd sat down in his office, the door having been so softly closed — Coleridge turned the knob to silence even the click — "is a little surgery. I've had a pain low down in my right side for a while now. The doctor wants to go in and, you know, take out a thing or two. Says he can do it the first day of vacation. So, it's a plan: I'll recuperate another several days or so, maybe a week and a half, and be back to school just after classes start up again."

ELFRIEDA AND I OCCUPIED THE waiting room together. Not exactly "together." She stood to one side, her arms folded over her bosom, solemnly, I thought, contemplating her husband's recovery at home. I sat reading a book. We had prayed with Coleridge before he was wheeled into surgery. For her that must have been enough togetherness.

An hour before the time estimated for the whole procedure, a doctor in hospital greens, his hair still covered, though he had removed his face mask, entered the room and turned to talk with us.

"Well. It isn't good news. The cancer — "

Cancer! Neither one of them had used that word before.

But I should have known.

"The cancer," said the doctor, "has metastasized. Mrs. Churchill, it has involved spleen, liver, kidneys — in one way or another, most of his abdominal organs."

He paused. He took on a patient, inquisitive expression, wait-

ing, I think, for the woman to ask a question or two. She didn't.
She kept her arms folded, and though her eyes had filmed somewhat, she kept her gaze on the doctor's face as well. Not in his
eyes. At the mask now ropy around his throat.

The pause stretched into an awkward length. The doctor ex-
changed his more compassionate expression for one concerned
with the business at hand. "I promise you," he spoke a perfunc-
tory promise, "we will do all we can. It isn't, well, the prognosis
isn't certain."

· Then, not shifting her eyes or herself Mrs. Churchill an-
nounced: "I will take him home today."

Even I knew the impossibility.

"Oh! Hmm. I'm sorry. We'll have to keep him here awhile.
Longer than awhile, I'm afraid. Yes. Longer."

LONGER THAN CHRISTMAS VACATION. ALMOST as long as the
month of January.

I visited him regularly. So did Elfrieda, of course, but not
always when I was there. When we did happen to arrive at the
same time, I saw how she had chosen to become a monument of
self-restraint. At my entering in she walked straight to the window, turned to peer out of it, whether into daylight or into darkness. The woman kept her arms folded fiercely across her chest.
Armor, I believe. An impenetrable breastplate.

Coleridge, on the other hand, received me with an open
kindness.

He would speak in that elemental murmur. Reduced to it, but melodious all the same.

Week after week the patient changed. His hair flattened upon the pillow. His cheeks grew gaunt and his eye sockets haunted. His teeth developed a yellow rime. He himself seemed to wither. And the color of his complexion changed into something drawn and dusty.

I would draw up a chair and sit by him. He appreciated the Psalms; not those that complained of sickness and enemies, but those that took comfort in the assurances of the shepherd.

Bless the Lord, O my soul,
  and all that is within me,
  bless his holy name.
Bless the Lord, O my soul,
  and forget not all his benefits—
who forgives all your iniquity,
  who heals all your diseases,
who redeems your life from the Pit,
  who crowns you with steadfast love and mercy,
who satisfies you with good as long as you live
  so that your youth is renewed like the eagle's.

"'As long as I live,'" he repeated. "And 'long' is the length of it. That's all. It is enough."

One afternoon shortly after the schoolchildren had raced into the streets for home, I approached the door to Coleridge's room, shrugging myself out of my overcoat. The door stood partly closed, but not completely. I slowed the approach, creeping forward, in order to peek in and decide whether I should go in or not.

Behind the door I saw Elfrieda, bent at her hips, leaning low over her husband. Lately he was sleeping most of the day. Pain medications put him out. And sometimes, because his eyes were half-lidded, the man seemed comatose.

Right now Elfrieda's face was inches above his. She was passing her left hand over his torso, flat open and so close to the sheets a waking man would have felt the heat. I'd never seen Elfrieda like this before. It caused a sweet melting in me, and an odd prickling behind my ears.

I must have made a little noise.

Elfrieda snapped upright, glanced at me in the doorway, then stomped to her position in front of the window, staring out in anger.

I despised myself for the intrusion. I would have left the hospital, except that soon I heard that deep, distant, rumbling thunder. His eyes still closed, Coleridge was laughing. He stretched his hand in my direction and crooked his fingers in invitation. Warily I stepped in.

And Coleridge began to speak.

"Oh, my wife, my wife." He opened his eyes. The whites had gone yellow, causing the pupils to seem almost golden. He gazed at the ceiling.

"I know what she wants. And I know what she needs. But I can't give it to her. Neither one."

Elfrieda didn't move. She gave no sign of hearing, not even the hunching of her shoulders—which might have indicated a severe resistance.

"I can't give it to her," he said in his most merciful voice. He reached for my hand and took it and drew me close to the bedside. "But I can give her the gettin'. Reverend. Pray with me."

We did. He chose the prayer by beginning it: "Our Father, who art in heaven; hallowed be thy name. Thy kingdom come …"

And so we prayed the Lord's Prayer all the way to the end. And together, scarcely audible, we whispered, "Amen."

In the few visitations that followed, Coleridge began to hiccup. Day and night.

THE DAY CAME WHEN, AGAIN, we were both in Coleridge's room, Elfrieda and I, each in our customary places, the window, the bedside chair.

Yes: there is a death rattle. It sounds like dry dice clattering behind the Adam's apple.

Elfrieda broke her pose. She whirled around and stared at me, wide eyed, uncertain. Suddenly she bolted around the bed. She faced Coleridge and stood wavering beside me. Then it was as if someone had taken a two-by-four and whacked her at the back of her knees: they broke. I mean that she dropped swiftly to the floor, grabbed her husband's enormous hands in hers—and all at once began to pray.

"Our Father who art in heaven! Hallowed be thy name! Thy kingdom come! Thy will be done on earth at it is in heaven!"

She pressed her face into Coleridge's shining palms. The prayer that had begun as a barked demand now softened. Could she smell her husband's scent? Did his great hands muffle her sterner tone?

"Give us this day our daily bread, and forgive us our trespasses ... as we forgive those who trespass against us. Lead us not," she dropped her voice to a murmur, "into temptation, but deliver us from evil.

"For thine is the kingdom. And the power. And the glory.

"Forever and ever. Amen."

When she had prayed the prayer to its end, Coleridge was dead.

She began gently to rock. But her face was still in his hands. She knew. There was no way that she couldn't have known. His spirit had gone from her.

I waited. Finally when I knew that she was not going to stand again, I moved to kneeling right behind her. I wrapped my arms around her shoulders and held her awhile.

Then I whispered directly into her ear: "Elfrieda, I have never seen a more glorious chariot to carry a soul to heaven than your prayer."

She began to shake with tears. It made me cry too.

She turned and embraced me too.

COLERIDGE CHURCHILL'S FUNERAL TOOK PLACE on January 29, 1981. He had been an important and well-respected man. Our little church was jam-packed with people black and white. Coats hunched end to end in every pew, like starlings cold on telephone wires.

Elfrieda and the two Churchill children sat in the first pew, right-hand side as you face the altar. They were adults, the son already teaching in northwestern Indiana. They were a family of honor, gracious in grief, reserving expressions of bereavement for times in private.

Through each of its ritual parts the service went well. Except when I said, "We pray the prayer our Lord taught us to pray—"

My back was turned to the congregation. I didn't see what happened next. But I heard it.

There came the harsh clicking of two heels on the floor, followed by the voice of a third-grade teacher.

She said: "We will *all* pray the prayer the Lord taught us to pray!"

So then I did look back at the congregation.

There stood Elfrieda Churchill. The only one standing, if you please. Confronting all the official and imposing folks and surveying them with a sharp eye to see whether anyone would contradict her:

"Our Father, who art in heaven!"

And so forth.

Letter #18

How long, good friends? How long since our last communication?

There's a reason why I haven't written another cancer letter for something like three months now. It would have focused mostly on varieties of pain without the authority or the urgency of an imminent death. Eternity would not have understructured my thought, granting it the value of spaciousness. Without these things, letters might have descended into a self-centeredness that invites nothing so much as pity — for until now we've had little new information regarding the cancer's progression within me.

Likely, the topic would have been: *I hurt. I hurt.*

Well, but this past autumn has been one of my more difficult seasons. I'll play the refrains: an increasing restriction of the air capacity of my lungs, which has necessitated my dragging oxygen canisters about with me; a dull whacklike bruising down my back and throughout my chest cavities; sharp whip-snap-pains in my left hip and thigh which, at sudden assertions, can cause me to gasp; those severe flulike symptoms, sweats, chills, a loathing of food, muscles gone to punk, which (if I hadn't known of the cancer) would have kept me home from teaching. And so forth and so on.

(Oh, forgive me these repetitions and the tired length of them. In several weeks it will have been a full year since I found that first mass in my neck. I'm constantly aware of these afflictions. But when I read them again from your points-of-view, they seem monotonous.)

Then, last month, the doctors ordered a series of tests: four CT scans, a pulmonary exam, blood work, a PET scan.

We saw our oncologists on the 10th and the 21st and then again, last week, the 28th of November.

While Thanne and I were driving to the chemical oncologist, we discussed my funeral. We discussed her plans for the years following my death (this is a common topic between us). We've begun to consult a lawyer regarding our will, and so are dealing with the thorny issue of my books, royalties, writings yet unpublished. This requires estate planning. And we need someone to take on the awful job of handling copyright determinations hereafter, the editing of the manuscripts I will not have revised — my papers, my archives. We've bequeathed early drafts of books, revisions, notes and researches applicable, as well as other relative documents to the library at Valparaiso University.

It hasn't been hard to talk about our will or what we want it to govern for a while after death. The generations after us will go on. The poet Richard Hugo published one of his later collections under the title *Making Certain It Goes On*. I know that urgency. I like the phrase. I've used it in these letters before. I consider it a pleasant responsibility.

Driving north to Chesterton we spoke in tones of the anteroom. All my symptoms had only been increasing. Ever since the battery of electronic examinations, we'd come to the conclusion (if not the conviction) that my only itinerary must be deathward.

I quoted for Thanne words which Dr. Jaroslav Pelikan uttered shortly before his own death:

If Christ is raised, nothing else matters. If Christ is not raised, nothing matters.

So we sat down before the physician, the young man with whom we've been consulting for a while now. He asked about my condition. Thanne and I scrolled through the points on our list. He listened, considered, thought, nodded. Then he began carefully to diagnose my difficult state. As before he allowed us to watch his thought processes while he walked through the possibilities—until he arrived at suggestions and prescriptions.

The pneumonitis has definitely taken over the top halves of my lungs, changing the cells into mere fibrous tissue incapable of transferring oxygen at all. And the condition was here to stay.

Whatever the radiation oncologist had said, ("Eighty percent of these cases clear up") the pneumonitis will dwell in my chest as long as I live. It acts within me as an inflammation, triggering broad varieties of hurt.

"Have you chosen," he asked me, "what to write in the time left?"

Put your affairs in order.

"Yes. I've started."

He suggested I struggle with less pure oxygen. It encourages the pneumonitis to spread even farther. I should walk. I should not worry about a hard racing of my heart. Working that organ won't damage it, but would rather strengthen it.

He wrote a prescription for ibuprofen to ease the inflammation. He required me to continue the morphine. In fact, it was doing good, nor did I feel any reaction except that, though the pain persisted, I could separate myself from it. I was taking warfarin as a blood thinner —

Then, in an off-handed subordinate clause, the doctor mentioned that he had found, in that battery of tests, no significant development of the tumors.

"*Wait a minute!* What did you say?"

The cancer itself was scarcely worse than it was three months ago. Not dormant, but the metabolism had slowed to a crawl.

But what about this pain?

It's real. But he couldn't identify the direct causes. People experience any number of different reactions to a continuing cancer.

"Don't stop working," he said. "Write."

Soon Thanne and I were sitting in the car that still sat in the clinic parking lot. How to assimilate the news. We fell into long pauses between sentences. What then? No funeral for a longer while than we'd thought? Time to do certain things yet? Planning is possible?

Life. Hum. We need to let the children know. What should we think, Thanne? What do *you* think?

A few days ago I finished a book regarding Leave-Takings without Home-Comings in this present life: from the parents, from the parents' house, from childhood, and so forth. Abraham from Haran, Jacob from Esau, Ruth from Moab, Christ from eternity— Matthew from us. I call it *Father and Son: Finding Home.* Essentially it tells the story of my thirty-six-year relationship with Matthew. Topics like this one no longer scare me: departures geographic, social, familial, spiritual—and this last for realms celestial.

Do you see why I have good reason to write you now? We've passed through an autumn of ignorance. There is news.

Soon enough this cancer will return and reclaim my attentions, drawing me back to the experiences of this last twelve-month. But I will live in the meantime. The Mean Time is remarkably short. I recognize this in all the fibers of my being, for these are they who have communicated corruption to me.

All the fibers of my being.

Perhaps that phrase may touch upon my reasons for refusing to use the imagery of warfare when speaking of my cancer. I have never construed my cancer as my enemy. No: please don't think I judge others who do (thoughtfully) choose the image, for whom "fighting" may be a helpful attitude. On the other hand I *am* critical of the media (and so much of the general populace) when, without genuine forethought, they routinely declare in their common parlance concerning a cancer death—or in their obituaries —that so-and-so has died after "a long battle with cancer."

Why does it always have to be a "battle"? What?—are folks fighting cancer good warriors if they win? (But what *is* winning?) Are they bad fighters, the unseated knights, if they lose? Die? Often the media's sentimentalized characterization is that it was a "heroic" battle. But few other personal failures are praised as "heroic." Those who fall in war. They are. But how often isn't this meant to varnish a failing campaign? Or, the reverse, to condemn the failing war that is eating up our men and women?

Cancer really isn't an issue of defeat or victory. We are all going to die: what a terrible, terribly total annihilation the language of warfare must make of our slaughters individual and wholesale, of our universal losses to sickness, disease, our wretched aggressions, the deaths of every human: *Hey ho! You lose!*—however we rouge the defeat by striving to ennoble it as "heroic."

Why not use the imagery that acknowledges how one truly experiences dying?—how one behaves in the face of death?—what one has to offer those who stand by in love and relationship? These considerations have been forms of discussion very familiar in the church of the past. Read Jeremy Taylor's meditations: *Holy Living and Holy Dying*. Before sciences and the medical profession began (if indirectly) to persuade us that cures could be possible for every disease we might diagnose, describe, explain and name; before commercials began to establish it as a principle that each affliction also had an antidote; before our society made "feeling good" an individual human right (setting at enmity anything that made us feel bad), we did not have so self-centered, so childish, so simplistic, unavailing and purposeless a frame of reference for the experience of sickness-unto-death.

For is it, in the end, *cancer* that we "battle"? I suggest that the true opponent isn't this condition, but that for which it stands: mortality. And if this observation is correct, then the foe has become some form of *God*. Him we "battle," right? But isn't Taylor's following portrayal truer and more consoling than to be destroyed by the Enemy Deity?

> Two differing substances were joined together with the breath of God, and when that breath is taken away, they part asunder and return to their several principles, the soul to God our Father, the body to the Earth our Mother; and what in all this is evil? Surely nothing, but that we are human; nothing, but that we were not born immortal, but by declining this change with great passion, or receiving it with a huge natural fear, we accuse the divine providence of tyranny, and exclaim against our natural constitution, and are discontent that we are human.

Or why not use the imagery of the psalmists in the Hebrew Scriptures? A human is his body or hers. (*Note:* even my use of possessive language here supposes a possessor of the body; which possessor, then [a mind? a soul?], is considered the "real" person.) But for the Hebrews the body/individual never exists in isolation (which is the result of our notion that the wholeness of a person *is* that person only). No, the "individual" exists always and only in relationships: to elements of creation; to a people, a tribe, a family; to God. Suffering a physical sickness is to experience the effects of a breakage in the body's significant relations. Sickness is not an enemy! It is a rooster's crow, calling me to the truth of myself and to the precise condition of my relationships — God, society, nature. Are there enemies? The psalmist knows some. Those who hate God. Those people(s) who attack him — yes, and who hurt the Lord in the attack; for wounding is distinguished from physical disease; but even human warfare and defeat are attributed to disobedience, our breaking of God's commandments and our breaking of the divine relationship. Rather than enemies, there is enmity.

Now they can use the language of "battle," where it is not a metaphor! Here it becomes the truth; but it isn't cancer which we battle. It is God and now *we* are the aggressors.

For my own part, I recognize cancer cells as parts of me (of Walt, the body-soul continuum). Cancer is tissue which is in company with all my other tissues — *all my fibers!* In company: even as my children are parts of our family (without whom the family itself would be something different). They (whether cells or kids) do become selfish, demanding more of family resources than other members can receive. But my children are not my enemy. And my diseases, far from acting the foe, are profound initiators of spiritual clarity, devout meditation, a faithful *(peaceful!)* seeking after God, praying, shaping thanksgivings for Jesus's rebuilding the pathways between God the Father and me. And just this (the reconciliation Christ has effected between the All-Father and all children) becomes the object of my most careful contemplations. And these contemplations are made more patient and more natural by the disease and by the convictions of mortality which the disease has infused in me.

The cancer, do you see, has accomplished a number of blessings for me.

But warfare, warfare, warfare has become so common a means to comprehend so many things: war on poverty, war on terror. We battle the statistics: for ratings, against competitors, for grades. We use the media as artillery by which to "get our message out," as opposed to getting ourselves into the shape the public requires. We fight (with grand "war chests") for victory in elections. (And then hope that our fightin' words can simply be puffed away as meaningless once this war is over. Bush: "I've been to the rodeo before." Well, how about a war on lying?) I believe that the narrowness of our interpretive constructs reveals the narrowness of our minds. More and more are our experiences bounded by verbal armories and the scopes of perpetual conflicts. We don't grow. How can we grow? Rather than permitting the interruptions of our familiar lives (like cancer) to enrich these lives, we impose old, timeworn patterns of thought upon the experience, reducing it and closing against us insight and discovery. Patterns which crush to a fine powder our adventures into the unknown. And so it is shaped to conform to — oh, I don't know — a schoolyard brawl, or the daily news. Nothing new. Nothing to call us into an ever newer light.

THANNE AND I ARE so grateful that you've accompanied us all this way: our tribe who bears with us the wayward choices of our cells as you would surely bear with us the wayward wanderings of our teenagers.

Were I to write these letters without others to receive them, they would lose dimension and resonance. But to write, as it were, before a chorus of ears and under a choir of minds — this grants me the sense of a surrounding congregation singing glory-hymns, yes, even now, right now, as I sit typing to you.

And as new news comes, I'll write again.

Walt

Letter #19

Dear Linda:

You will remember the first day of our Liturgics class last August. The fall semester. Days steaming with the heat. It seems to me long ago. I had decided to be direct about my cancer before my students. I didn't want folks to tiptoe around the professor nor to be distracted from the project at hand, which was learning. Without sentiment, then, mildly and clinically, I described my condition.

You cried.

I saw it.

Not right then, but weeks later, you chose to walk back to my office with me. After class you had piddled with your books and notes until we alone were left in the room. I could assume it was natural that you fell into step with me. I was pulling that canister of oxygen behind me — the outward sign of things internal.

"How do you —" you started to say. You were searching for the right approach. Then: "What do you think? I mean, that you're so close to dying, how do you handle it? What do you do?"

We wore jackets. At least I did, against the chill breezes. My body had begun to feel as chilly as the weather was hot. I couldn't get myself warm again.

You remember the answer I gave you. I know you do. Anyone who takes notes during the sermons I preach — she retains particulars. She doesn't forget.

I said, "I hold death lightly in my hands." I opened the flats of my two palms, then lifted them up and down, the left one down, the right one up, and so forth, making the motion of a balance. "Life or death. Either one is a gift to me. I don't yearn for one over the other."

What I told you that day was true. And you seemed satisfied by the answer.

Since then, though, I've continued to probe the thing. Why *am* I so cavalier about matters so grave? What grants me freedom from anxiety? How can I explain this to others? To you, Linda. I owe you more than my immediate mood. What good can it do you if I don't offer you more than "I'm fine." "*I* am fine" proves nothing more for you than that fineness is possible in the face of death.

So, then: How does this peace come about?

If you don't mind, I'll be your teacher again, developing the nature of my peace by references to the Bible.

It's a lesson. Therefore I beg your patience.

Remember that in the Gospel of John, Jesus raises Lazarus by calling out, *Lazarus, come forth!* Remember, too, that when Mary Magdalene is suffering death (both her Lord's and so her own) Jesus brings her back to life by saying one word only: *Mary.*

Linda, my dear student and my friend: it's in the naming.

Skip with me among a few Old Testament events.

Genesis 1:1 – 2:23

AT THE CREATION, THE LORD God spoke not one, but two sorts of languages.

There was the utterance of pure creation. God's words *were* the thing that had not existed before he called it out of nothing. *Let there be light!* This wasn't a command, that light should be formed to obey and come rushing to the Creator. Light was not, nor *is* not, like flaming horses galloping Godward from the caves of nothingness. Nor did this language work (first) like a blueprint, a design according to which (later) the Father constructed light.

Rather let me draw for you a fanciful image to come near to the quality of God's creating language. As little children might, imagine God as a body with a mouth. Anthropomorphize the deity. Now then, see God open up his splendid gap, and *see* the creating word and the created thing at once: see Light come flooding from God's mouth. *That* is the word, *and* that is the thing. They are one. This is the language which the Creator reserves for himself only. No one else could ever utter such a speech.

On the other hand, at creation the mighty Lord God spoke a second sort of language. This was the language of naming things already created. Having created the light, its opposite was brought into existence: darkness. God separated the two so that they kept replacing one another (for this was also the creation of Time). But listen: *God called the light "Day," and the darkness he called "Night."*

It was the same with the firmament: *"God called the dome Sky."*

The gathered waters below were named *"Sea."*

The dry land, *"Earth."*

It was this second language which the Lord God gave to humanity to speak.

Out of the ground the Lord God formed every animal of the field and every bird of the air, and brought them to the man to see what he would call them. And whatever the man called a living creature, that was its name.

Please, one more thought about this kind of Naming:

Each name was not merely a handle for the clay object created. It was not a referent mentally pointing to the thing.

No. Naming in the Hebrew Scriptures was an event. It acted on the thing named, working three changes.

I. That it was given a name brought it out of the darkness of unknowing. We could not *know and discuss* the created thing without knowing the name that revealed it to us. By its name it entered our vocabulary—and so our knowing.

2. It established for the thing created a *relationship* with every other named thing. Think in terms of words (names) as they are

used in a sentence. The noun is no longer alone, but has its place in the order of that sentence, a relationship, community. So it is for all things.

3. And the name often declared the *purpose* of its existence. *Israel, you will be for me a kingdom of priests.* Priesthood in and for the world is a marvelous, even a divine, reason for being. Naming saved us from the hell of uselessness.

Remember now the creative power of the naming of an animal, pieces of the cosmos.

Genesis 32:22–32

HERE IS THE STORY OF Jacob's wrestling with an "Angel" all night long—a mighty engagement between two Titans, one an ancestor of a people, the other the presence of God. Guess which must win?

But listen again to a brief conversation that takes place in the midst of such striving:

He said to him, "What is your name?"

And he answered, "Jacob."

The name means something like *treacherous usurpation*: Jacob had stolen his brother's birthright and his blessing. He had even tricked his uncle in order to obtain a good portion of Laban's wealth. The name revealed its bearer.

Then his almighty opponent said, *"You shall no longer be called 'Jacob,' but Israel. For you have striven with God and with your own kind, yet you have prevailed."*

By the changing of his name, God changed his being, his character and relationships and purpose. Israel means something like, *The one who strives with God,* which may be taken as a pun. He has always striven against God, even when he seemed to be striving with Esau and Laban and others. But now and hereafter his striving will be on behalf of God!

Exodus 3:4

WHEN THE LORD GOD CALLS Moses by his name, *"Moses, Moses!"* the shepherd answers: *"Here I am."* However common such a response was in those days, it manifests a sweet declaration by the human: I dwell in this relationship. I abide in your voice by the calling of my name, for I abide in the name. In your presence it *is* me.

Call his name and Moses whole exists in that utterance of God.

John 1:42

[ANDREW] BROUGHT SIMON TO JESUS, who looked at him and said, "You are Simon son of John. You are to be called Cephas" (which is translated "Peter").

Consider the change Christ's word effects for and in his "Rock."

John 10

AND HERE, LINDA, COMES THE real source of my peace on the threshold of death.

Watch in this chapter for the relationship between the Holy Shepherd and his flock:

The sheep hear his voice. He calls his own sheep by name and leads them out. When he has brought out all his own, he goes ahead of them, and the sheep follow him because they know his voice. They will not follow a stranger, but they will run from him because they do not know the voice of strangers.

It is in the voice of the shepherd that the sheep (twice promised) find assurance and protection. Moreover, by that voice the shepherd calls each sheep by name. What does this "calling the sheep his own by name" accomplish?

Read on:

I am the good shepherd. I know my own and my own know me, just as the Father knows me and I know the Father. And I lay down my life for the sheep. I have other sheep that do not belong to this fold. I must bring them also, and they will listen to my voice.

There is that voice again, and by it we (who are the other sheep that the Lord will bring in) will know the Lord and his dying on our behalf.

Again, the fourth reference to this powerful voice:

My sheep hear my voice. I know them, and they follow me. I give them eternal life, and they will never perish. No one will snatch them out of my hand. What my Father has given me is greater than all else, and no one can snatch it out of the Father's hand. The Father and I are one.

And this, finally, is the merciful consequence of the Savior's calling our names. Eternal life!

Linda, how did Jesus raise Lazarus, whom he dearly loved, from the dead? He called the dead man by his name! *Lazarus!*

And how did he revive Mary Magdalene, grieving the death of her whole existence? *Mary.*

So it shall be with me.

WHEN I COME TO DIE, what must be my immediate state? (I can hardly call it "my experience," for how can one-who-is-not experience his not-ness. All the engines and impressions of experience itself are shut down.) My state then must be that of one dismantled. Of one gone through rot, a depersonalized soup. What God created degenerates into the un-creation which existed before my birth. I anticipate, then, a state of knowing nothing, for the capacity *to know* at all has passed away—and with it the knower, me.

But then the creating Word (whose flesh as mine was once annihilated) will come to the Absence which is the not-me—and utter a creating word. In that second language which the Creator used at the Creation, that dazzling *naming* of things will Jesus speak.

The divine Word which (as with Jacob) remakes folks by naming them with a new name, that Word will also come for me.

The shepherd will come—he who leads me out by my name and by the resounding gift of his voice.

And he will say to my dead self: *Walter!*

And I will be again.

The creating word itself will give me ears to his voice. And a mind of soaring mystery to know it. And I like Lazarus will rise.

I, like Mary Magdalene, will emerge from the death of hopelessness and anguished tears and distress.

"Walter," Jesus will say, and in that instant my soul will know Jesus, that it is he. And in the light of his familiar voice — in the sweet re-declaration of my name — I will even know me, who I am, and therefore *that* I am!

Mary cried, "I have seen the Lord!" But I will cry: *I am seeing the Lord right beside me. Oh you heavens, I am Moses, for in God's calling me by name, I am empowered to answer, "Here I am!"*

Resurrected, do you see?

Right now, therefore, I am to hold lightly both death and life — and the life which shall be.

Linda, be at peace in your place across the waters. New Guinea. Being a stranger for a while has nothing to do with one's final arrival with Christ. The sheep upon his dear shoulders cannot be a stranger, but homing and home at once.

As for me, I don't pray for death. But I wouldn't mind an early visitation. Forgive me this next complaint: there is just so much about this world and its leaders which is so disappointing. It crushes my heart. And prospects that have withered, and fame which itself draws the enmity that deflates the famous, and such wretched, wretched, stupid, arrogant, self-aggrandizing leadership! How they mishandle the world! Industry has no soul. It works toward its own health and growth, its own self, period! It will do anything to forestall its own death, raising the wave upon which its voracious captains rise and arise!

I long for the righteousness of the king described in Isaiah 11.

But I need not think of death always as an escape. I may, after all, depart in the peace that you and others give me. See? You represent a host of the gracious by whom the world may be saved. And my children and my grandchildren will find good hearts among whom to make their home.

I believe that, for the sake of the righteous in this world—however few they may be—God does not destroy the world. It is a comfort. I do not need to fight forever. I can sleep.

Walt

A Fifth Meditation:
If I Thought Anything,
I Thought, "Cheek"

......

LET ME TELL YOU A little story of a little resurrection which was like the final one to come.

Late in the winter of 1982 (twenty-seven years ago) the doctors X-rayed my chest and found dark spots on the lower lobe of the right lung. They couldn't read it absolutely as a series of tumors, so they scheduled me for a bronchoscopy. An outpatient procedure. They would run a tiny, tiny video camera and pincers up through my nose, down my throat and through my bronchial tubes until they reached that deep place of suspicious spots.

Under bright lights in an examination room they prepared me by spraying a local anesthetic on the back of my throat. "Numb the gag reflex," Dr. Wadell said.

So the narrow cord went up and down and through. The intrusion was a rough presence on the move.

But before they could reach the target area, the head of this slender device broke through the soft tissue, causing blood to fill the lungs. Spontaneously I began a hoarse huffing, as if to cough up the fluid. But the cord kept my larynx open, and the liquid was too deep to bring up. Sitting on the side of the metal examination table, I started to panic. I couldn't cry it aloud, but I screamed it in my mind: *I'm drowning!*

They withdrew the tiny camera and the tiny nipper that had gone down for tissue to biopsy.

Dr. Wadell said: "We shouldn't take chances with this."

He recommended surgery — a thoracotomy. They would open my chest and retract the ribs on my right side in order to remove that lowest lobe of my right lung.

"Get ready for a long convalescence."

"How long?"

"If all goes well, six weeks."

Nevertheless, we agreed, Thanne and I.

ON THE DAY OF THE surgery, good friends accompanied Thanne. I was wheeled down the hallway as she walked beside me. We held hands. Our children were twelve and eleven and nine and eight years old. I thought of them. I went feet-first through cream-colored swinging doors: *Surgery #3.*

The night before my hospitalization, I'd sat in the center of my study. Slowly I moved my eyes over the spines of all the books shelved before me. So many unread. I lived in the promise of reading these. All of them containing plans for future writings. I sat, trying to understand a great gaping hole in that future.

"Walt? Can you count backward for me? Count backward from one hundred."

Soon, then, the end of consciousness, the end of memory. I entered an early unknowing.

After I'd fully awakened again, more than twenty-four hours after the surgery, Thanne told me what had happened in my absence.

When Dr. Wadell reported to her in the waiting room that everything had gone well, Thanne's comforters prayed, then left.

She remained in the room alone, wondering whether to stay (as she wished) or to go home and get some sleep (as the nurses wished for her).

In an hour or two the decision was made.

A nurse rushed in to say that I had become a "bleeder." I was bleeding into my abdomen. They had to open my chest again and find the vessel and cauterize it. The surgeon would return as soon as things were stable.

But it was late when the news came that I was once again in Recovery. My arms taped to flat boards so that I wouldn't tear out the tubes and the monitors.

I knew none of this at the time. There was *no* knowing until the second or the third day (I can't remember which).

I recall dwelling in a sort of dream of darkness: a being without form or shape, a consciousness drawn down to a pinpoint.

AND THEN THIS: I FELT the (re)creation of my cheek. A warm sensation was actually granting shape to my cheek. If I thought anything, I thought: *Cheek.* And then: *My cheek.* A new creation!

Next I was given a forehead. Then eyelids (closed, sightless); a chin and jaw; then, by a sudden fire, the back of my hand.

I built the rest of me from these several attributes. And then I realized how the pieces of myself had come again to be.

Thanne was sitting in the darkness beside me. She had been caressing me with her hand: my cheek, my forehead, and the rest of it. And I, like the baby waking to the universe, had not thought, *Hand.* Did not think *the loving touching of my wife.* That hand didn't exist. But its benefits did. I knew the benefits before I knew their cause. I knew my self before I could reflect on the relationship that had renewed that self.

I wonder whether this isn't the way babies become conscious of the world, first by sensing and considering the *self* its parents communicate to it by stroking, embracing, nursing.

I wonder whether this isn't the way the dead come to life, caressed by the palpable love of Jesus.

Letter #20

March 4, 2007

I'M BEGINNING TO THINK OF myself as a reporter in the messy, inchoate, much unobserved front, sending messages back to those who will, sooner or later, follow. And if the simile holds up, then it is required of me to maintain the gaze long after shelling and the immediate bleeding are past — watching a slower-motion fallout, lingering through changes in the weather ... or slow-healing, long-term wounds (let us say, wounds of the deep, psychological, or else of the out-patient-at-Walter-Reed variety.)

All right. Let's say that the reporter is indeed conscientious. How much more must he depend upon readers who can also find value in reportage which persists long past white heat and dramatic violence! The media isn't terribly interested in what's lukewarm and nuanced, un-fierce, un-tensioned — though this is not altogether that. No, this contains its own compacted violence.

You, friends. You, my family abroad:

It is for you I write, under your interest I persist in closely observing even now — and finding (on your account) insights I would not have been patient enough to wait for ante cancer. Hence: my dispatches, letters from the land of cancer.

Another level of trouble bedevils the afflicted whose illness persists not months but years. I speak for many, many people who may not necessarily die of the sickness they suffer, but whose suffering can often outlast the identifying specific symptoms and effects of the sickness.

I find myself exhausted. Endlessly. There is always the physical exhaustion — but that draws upon other, necessary energies, causing also a psychological exhaustion, and yet further sorts of exhaustion which I cannot classify.

Please hold that thought a moment.

When I am strong I am generally a good person because I truly *want* to be good. Wit and health and guilt and a genuine kindness are my means for controlling the more selfish, even malicious, tendencies in my nature. Yes, I do mean the "Old Adam" in me — but I do not want that understood as a vague mistake in the human genome, a flaw of the species. No, there are very particular behaviors of evil in my spirit, deviances peculiar to my character, a pitiful, cowardly sort of arrogance, an inability to let go of small aggravations, a peevish desire for revenge. And so forth. I belong to the human race indeed. (And so I inherit sinfulness.) But these behaviors belong to me! (And so I sin.) And I know them. And when I am not tired, I can control their outward, public manifestations.

But these long exhaustions of my long disease disable me. I lose the strength for restraint.

The "troubles" which this releases are not restricted to me alone. The unregarded sin, the uncontrolled trespass (the lion let out of the zoo barred by my will-toward-goodness) attacks my friends and my family and my wife. And then it is these, oh, my most beloved, who suffer. My conduct of unkindness strips me bare and isolates me and can undermine my better reputation with a worser truth. There. That, besides the levels of lingering exhaustions, is the worst extent of my "trouble." But the "troubles" dealt to the undeserving! The persistent complaints and brooding dissatisfactions with which I meet their grace and sympathy (which renders them the more vulnerable) — these are caustic wounds, blindsiding wounds, baffling wounds difficult to heal, O Lord, my guilt and my grief.

And then — recognizing the consequences of the Old Adam's liberation — I must, I must, I absolutely *must* believe in the mercy of God which makes merciful the people whose mercy I do dearly need. And this is what forgiveness looks like to me: that those I wounded are healed in the name of Jesus....

Suddenly three weeks ago my brother, Michael John Wangerin, died. He made his home in Denver, Colorado. He died in

Colorado Springs, at our parents' house. He was fifty-eight years old. He desired death.

As soon as my family learned of my cancer, it was Mike who called me before any other sibling, parent, cousin.

His first words, graveled by his own weariness, were: "I'm sorry, Wally. But you know, don't you? It should be me."

Jealous of my terminus!

I know Mike. I've known his character and its complexities ever since his baptism. In fact, his is the first baptism I can visually remember. He was an infant of devastating grace and beauty, black-brown pupils, and flashing eyes, and a dimpled smile of the love of living, his skull, brow and face shaped as finely as a porcelain ewer. There was nothing bruised nor squashed about this baby. A little man as medieval painters once painted Jesus, proportioned like a little man standing on Mary's knee.

Before my heart's eye it is not just the fifty-eight-year-old man, this lithe and weary soul, who died. It is also that winsome boy. It's the vibrant child who first entered Virginia Park Elementary School in Edmonton, the fourth of four boys, eager to join his elder brothers in walking to and fro the school, in reading and learning, and in this: entering the whole wide world together. Brotherhood! His was a laughing face. Every Christmas our mother bought all four of us matching flannel shirts. Mike delighted more than any of us in the symbol of solidarity.

But then that first-grader ran into difficulty, especially in reading. In those days his disability was not understood, went undiagnosed. Dyslexia was interpreted as laziness. It came of a contrarian nature, so people thought, of a stubborn disobedience, a refusal to *try!* Then it was—all the way back then—that my brother began to die. Scorned and scourged for what he couldn't help. Scolded into his own convictions of unworthiness. I can recall the fourth-grader curled up, lying on his side under the dining room table and crying and pleading, "Leave me alone. Leave me alone."

Strikingly beautiful, dark eyed, naturally athletic.

He went to Viet Nam. He laid his later anguish to the jungles of that disconsolate war.

But he married wonderfully. He reentered the child's life of laughter and of gratitude.

Once I said to him, "What changed you?"

He said, "Love."

"Yes," I said. "That Kathy loves you."

"No," he said. "That I love Kathy."

They bore three sons. And these had shining eyes. And one grandson of deep dimples, and another burbling up a curdled milk—that last child coming shortly before he died. And it was an abiding misery wore him out. Ah, my brother!

But then death came exactly three weeks ago. It was all my Mikes that died that night. And all his dyings that came to an end. A sort of whipsawing, knowing as much as I knew of my brother all the years of his life—how little was his fault, but how much he bore the fault; and during the last years he felt so compelled to serve, but service under his circumstances crushed him. So ungratefully received. Beautiful boy! Youth, man: all of this dying. All of this still living in my heart now, strained as wide as Canaan.

Oh, my Love! Your love ignited. Love exacerbated. Love reaching and not finding. Love so hot with the purity of its loving that it scorches more than itself, scorches my small emotional reserves, my poor wit, my slender will.

My grief, so intense it takes my breath away.

Weak, I am the further weakened.

Weakened, I am the less capable of keeping the lion under control, or the roaring of Adam housed. And because of a headlong love, I sin the more. No, this is no way to reverence my brother. No. And I am so much the sorrier.

On the other hand, I have not once grieved over *my* dying. Never. I approach its completion with an equanimity that permits these present days to be as productive and as filled with detail and experience as any other days I've lived here below.

There, this I beg of heaven: strengthen me, O Lord, in all my weaknesses. Strengthen my faith, that the Spirit's peace which eases my death yet to come might also ease my grief for my brother's death.

Forgiveness. Let forgiveness be the healing of those I've hurt. That, my God, is evidence even for the blind.

Call my brother Michael by his name.

Walt

Letter #21

June 6, 2007

Friends in the Gaps as well as the Letters:

Yesterday, Tuesday, a CT scan. Today I am eating strawberries. Next Tuesday I'll sit with my separate oncologists and read the scans of yesterday.

The strawberries!

Without having spoken to one another regarding the picking and the consuming of the fat, sweet fruit of our raised strawberry bed, Thanne and I enjoyed precisely the same gratitude for precisely the same grace.

Perhaps you recall my contemplations while planting this bed a year ago, recorded in a Cancer Letter of that period. I had built the frame of cedar wood, then filled it with a mixture of a good soil purchased and our own field-dirt. Last May I planted six sets at easy distances one from the others. All through the summer I pinched the white five-petaled flowers and the tiny, hard, green, emerging fruits so that each plant would put its energies into roots and runners and a green leafy growth. While I knelt at the bed, pinching the pretty heads, I couldn't shake a sort of cosmic question:

What of the yield? Who will pick my ripe red berries in the year when I'm not here to know or else to testify to the pleasure of the planting? Who will eat the fruit of my present labors?

That unanticipated year is this year. And behold: I am permitted to close a cycle of life, intensely sensitive to the simplicity of its round, unvarnished shape—and to the grace of it. It's *me! I'm* the one eating the fruit of my own labors! I haven't died. Thanne and I and those we love, we feed from the bed my hand had planted.

The contemplations of the planter a year ago have grown the more complex, embracing the First Creator who keeps on re-creating:

> What thou givest us, we gather; thou openest thine hand, and we are filled with good things. Thou hidest thy face, we are troubled; thou takest away our breath [our lungs' breath!], we die and return to the dust. Thou sendest forth thy breath [the Almighty's breath!] and we are created, and thou renewest the face of the earth.

My grandchildren, who last year knew me bald, will gather this summer around their planting papa, whose head is a curly mop, as wild as the vines in our strawberry bed, thick and given to bowing before the holy winds. Why, my everlasting straight hair has come in wavy—oh, you rake! How your wife loves to caress it.

My grandchildren will eat some of the eight pints of strawberry jam I put up five days ago. All comes around. And the coming-around of a single year of berries and babies signifies the coming-around of life to Life again: the harvest of God the Planter and Picker, the gracious Ingatherer. *Ahhh.*

THIS, THEN, YESTERDAY:

I dressed in a T-shirt and sweatpants which I bound to my body by rope alone. I fasted. I presented myself to radiology at 2:30 in the afternoon, filled out (those everlasting) forms, signed papers, was led into the room of a looped machine, where I fixed myself prone upon a hard, narrow, vinyl plank. I obeyed the technicians. I raised my arms. I found two handles behind my head and gripped them and waited to hear the order refusing me breath. My metal plank like a tongue, together with my whole corpus, was sucked swiftly into the round maw of the machine.

A short breath. Hold it....

But I have so little breath to hold....

In a smooth movement—but abrupt enough to turn my body into cargo—the tongue began to carry me out again.

When can I exhale and breathe?

When I was in high school I could swim underwater back and forth in an Olympic pool four lengths long. Without coming up for air. Now I can scarcely walk without *stopping* twice each length to woof in fresh air. If my breath is taken away from me, as the psalmist says (even for good reasons, to diagnose the activities of my cancer) I will die.

This procedure, not in itself disturbing or painful, is the computerized axial tomography which keeps me humble and dependant. (Breathe, O Lord, that I might breathe.)

Next week we will read the results.

I am bound to be honest in all things regarding this experience. So this next is another confession: I still do approach these doctors' visits with apprehension. It is four months since the last visit which I detailed for you, wherein Thanne and I received (all unexpectedly) the good news of the slow growth and near inactivity of my tumors. Never mind that. Lately my chest has rumbled and cracked at every breath exhaled. There is some sort of thickish fluid in there, deeper than the small packets of my sucked-in wind can plumb: so I cough and cough, ever renewing the itch which keeps renewing the cough — but which my pitiful efforts cannot reach to scratch. Cycling downward. Squeezing my lungs like an accordion on a poor chord, until not a bubble of air is left in me.

So I grow apprehensive of what we might find in me.

THANNE AND I HAVE TALKED at length about my burial. What will we do with this standing dust once it has failed? Where shall we lay it?

I'm no longer able to give bits of it away. Corneas, skin, a heart or a liver. Cancer disqualifies me. There is no need to preserve it for the sake of others.

We can't imagine the purpose of caskets and vaults and plots with comforting views — not, at any rate, when the cost of such elaborate dying saps value from the living family.

Abraham at last was "gathered to his people." This wasn't a reference to resurrection, since in those days resurrection wasn't a concept. Life continued after death in the lives of one's descendants. What was gathered to his people were his bones. His corpse was laid in a cave where bodies rotted away to the bones alone. These dry bones next were gathered together with the bones of his wife — and with bones of an Israelite's ancestors after that people had lived long in their land; then all the bones were deposited into a small depression near the back of the cave.

Such a burial was not much different in Jesus's day.

Even our medieval ancestors, who *did* anticipate a resurrection, were buried whole with the notion that at the last day their spirits would return and animate again the clay that once was them before corruption.

But martyrs were burned without the fear that their dust might not again be found at the great getting-up day.

How the body is laid "to rest" is governed more by our cultures than by any directive of our religion.

I will be cremated. We both will be, Thanne and I.

But we do recognize the value of a place where those who love us might come and physically direct their sorrows and then their own joys in life. So we choose not to scatter my ashes, but to put them into the ground: earth to earth, after all (which committal otherwise becomes a fiction in these days when rules and regulations demand sealed vaults for the human body, while animal bodies, however infected, are indeed laid naked in the ground, becoming ground).

For Thanne's sake after I die (for mine if she precedes me), and for the sakes of our children, we've tried to figure what sort of place might satisfy their reasons for returning. The ashes of our sister-in-law were poured into the ground of a garden beside her church. We saw how her husband would sit in that garden and mourn, and then as time passed, meditate. What a genial surrounding. A garden. Eden. The garden near Calvary, where Joseph of Arimathea's tomb received that body of our Lord.

A garden, then.

A garden close to the place where our children grew up. A garden already devoted to worship. Ground consecrated.

UNTIL THEN I MURMUR PSALM 104 more devoutly than before my lungs turned fibrous with the pneumonitis that will (we know now) attend me for the rest of my days:

> *When you take away their breath, they die and return to their dust.*
> *When you send forth your breath, they are created. . . .*
> *I will sing to the Lord as long as I live*
> *I will sing praise to my God while I have being. . . .*

A Sixth Meditation:
I Will Never Plant
a Seed in You

......

WHEN I WAS A CHILD and played in the dust of the summer, running through woods and patches of sunlight, it was the scent on the backs of my arms I loved most to smell.

I'd snuffle that skin below my nose. I would let my own humidity release the brown, dry, mossy scent, and close my eyes a moment. Leatherlike skin: it smelled of the soil cupped among the brutal tree roots; smelled of briar twigs and rabbit fur; of the stiff rustlings of the lilac bush; of bird feathers flattened upon the leaf-mold ground. The wings of finches smearing the sky. A puff-burst, a cough of blue spores. The pollen-thick air and solitary bumblebees.

My flesh and the creatures of all creation, made one.

I ran among—I ran beneath and upon—the stuff of which my running was made. An animal communion.

What did I have to fear? There were no parents in the fields. No one to scold me into an imprisonment of my body, sole and alone. Shame had been a burning isolation. Classroom scorn for my ineptitude. The offending lassitude of daydreaming (*I can't help it, I promise, I promise!*), but criminal and selfish nonetheless. The boy who lay on the floor behind the radio, his chin on his fist, gazing at bright filaments in their vacuum tubes and imagining the lights of whole cities therein, the boy soon whacked on his back for indolence. Contempt and criticism and punishments were my human community's rejection of the Wally-self until (as the mystic says) I had became "a nothing in a nowhere."

Running in the woods over bracken and the carpet of old leaves blackening; watching for black raspberries at the edges of clearings and pulling the fruit-like caps from their small waxy-bald heads: I am vines and trees and roots and earth and the fruit I eat.

I am summer.

Letter #22

August 10, 2007

Gentle Souls and Merciful Spirits All:

Time used to tumble for me. Like the mountain stream that breaks at the big rocks, spouts and plunges at speed from crags to canyons. Time was narrow, then, and very fast.

Now Time has slowed to a stately progression. I measure it in day/feet — feet per day. For there are fewer days left to me and heavier feet for the passage. Slowth: it requires enormous patience. Slowth: a damming up of an accumulated anxiety. The consequence of a body restrained, slower than an infant's crawl. My motion by disease reduced to the child's eternal wait for good things far away.

On the other hand, slowth is no trouble at all. Where once

Time tumbled, now Time has widened. Like the river that covers a broad plain. And the patience I thought was severity has become my benefaction.

I don't look forward so much any more, dashing to grasp the future. I look left and right. I've the Time, you see, to scrutinize all that *is*. And what *is* companions me. The trees can't lift their roots and move. A single motion fills a season. Well, then: let me abide by them awhile. My toes, my roots. A good rain can linger almost forever.

The shorter my Time, the vaster my scope.

Oh, my beautiful granddaughter! What you are right now doesn't need a future to give it purpose or fullness, or to make the present girl a better one. You are! You are, you are — and for me it is enough. Sure, you may marry one day. Will I be there to kiss you? Right now I don't know. But now I don't beg for that particular piece of future, nor do I bargain for it. Child, you are! And I am. And I have the Time to let the whole of you fill the whole of my Now.

This, girl: just this. Tip of my finger to the tip of yours. It is altogether enough.

Let me illustrate the pragmatic benefits of patience.

For years before cancer broke the speed of my Time and spread its silver motion as far as the horizons, I never took my socks off. Well, not my right sock. Under the nail of that great toe (concealed) was a fungus that blackened the length and breadth of it. I'd heard somewhere that smearing Vicks VapoRub over the nail day after day could kill the fungus and return the toe to its former health—and me to my former purity.

I tried the trick. Fairly often at first, sitting on the side of my bed, my right ankle upon my left knee, applying the goo with the flat of my thumb. But in those days Time kept catching me up and rushing me straightway into the headwaters of my days. Narrow spout, hurtling stream, my paper boat breathless upon its back, now, Now! I had no Time, no leisure to attend to the toe. *Years,* I say: black as compost.

But cancer cut the speed, enforced a more casual floating, and opened an eternity between my shower and my breakfast.

If I could take interest in a gradual sunrise, well, I could in my person mimic that solar motion and—what is just as interesting—rub the Vicks slowly, deeply into the nail now softened by warm tub-water.

And I know you know how slowly the nail on the great toe grows. In a month I noticed that the fungus, like a black window shade, was rising. The long morning of the black sun!

And it has arisen. And every Time I trim the nail, I razor away another slice of black.

Cancer has cured me.

Soon I'll remove the right sock too.

SURELY IT'S HIGH TIME—isn't it?—that we pay as much attention to the blessings of a long affliction as we do to the pain for which we curse it. Please: it's not a man's peculiar interpretation or a woman's particular gift for longsuffering patience which enables each to live the sickness better than another person does. It's a faith available to everyone. (Though there always is, of course, a learning curve.)

Pay attention!

In the Lakota tongue: *wachin ksapa yo!* — whose meaning is closer to "Be attentive" than to something we do sporadically. Be ever in the state of attention.

For the footfall of an ant may be as thunderous as a maverick at full gallop, and as meaningful as the sky.

Rather than drowning awareness, or drugging it, or shrouding ourselves in pity or a persistent sorrow, consider companionship: the tree that waits upon our own slowth in order to befriend us. The wren who, quick as wit, follows ever her singular path and by her repetitions sticks in the same familiar places in Time. The child whose entire life is caught up in a minute which is as long as a lifetime.

The toenail healed in Slow Time. The fullness of experience between the shower and a cup of coffee.

Walt

A Seventh Meditation:
Bright as Crystal

......

THE ANGEL SHOWED ME THE river of the water of life, bright as crystal, flowing from the throne of God and of the Lamb, flowing through the middle of the street of the city.

On either side of the river is the tree of life with its twelve kinds of fruit, yielding month by month another fruit.

And the leaves were for the healing of the nations.

HE WHO TESTIFIES TO THESE things says, "Surely, I come quickly."

Amen. Come, Lord Jesus.

Walter Wangerin, Jr.

Postscript

April 15, 2008

STABLE. MY TUMORS SLEEP. THE earth turns. My Lord is near. I
am quiet here — and stable.

Walter Wangerin Jr

Father and Son

Finding Freedom

Walter Wangerin Jr, National Book AwardWinning Author, and Matthew Wangerin

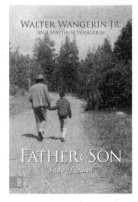

"Given our history, this father and this son might well have gone completely separate ways .... And only in becoming a father did I even begin to understand what it meant, what it was, what would be required of me, and who I was/am within that identity, father."

Pastor, author, and father Walter Wangerin Jr., along with his adopted son, Matthew, tell the story of their own lifelong relationship and how they survived times when brokenness and bitterness seemed inevitable. It is the story of Matthew's desperate search for independence and his father's own search for authentic fatherhood.

This is a book of deep emotion and serious meditation about broken lives and redemption. *Father and Son* weaves together each writer's personal story and shows how earthly fathers and sons are shaped by a Creator's relationship with his creation, and how within the human experience of parenting we discover insights into the spiritual nature of home, family, and eternity itself.

Together, father and son have written a book that must be experienced as well as read. It's a book parents will want to bring their lives to, not just their attention. *Father and Son* is the story of all of us, for we are all wayward children in need of a loving, patient father.

Hardcover, Jacketed: 978-0-310-28394-2

Jesus

Walter Wangerin Jr.

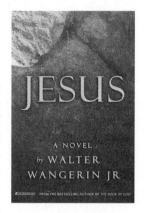

With eloquence and beauty, the award-winning author of *Book of the Dun Cow*, *The Book of God*, and *Paul: A Novel* turns his pen to history's most compelling figure: Jesus of Nazareth. In vibrant language, Walter Wangerin Jr. sweeps away centuries of tradition and reveals a man of flesh-and-heart immediacy. Passionate, intelligent, and irresistibly real, this is a Jesus pulsing with life who will captivate you as thoroughly as he did the men and women who walked with him across Galilee's golden countryside.

Days of centuries past become today, lit with bright colors of the imagination. Wangerin shows you Jesus through the eyes of the two people who were with him at very the foot of the cross, the two who knew and loved him best: the beloved apostle, and Jesus' mother, Mary.

Here is a magnum opus of image and emotion: Jesus bringing his father the sacrificial lamb in Jerusalem's temple . . . Mary desperately searching for her son in the wind-lashed rain . . . the cry of gratitude from a leper's lips . . . the loving intimacy of Jesus in prayer . . . the fury of religious leaders . . . the agony of an iron crucifixion spike piercing human sinew . . .

Loving son, intimate friend, and brilliant teacher, tender in heart, fierce in anger, wholehearted in joy and in grief, deeply human yet unmistakably divine—this is the Jesus who lives and breathes in these pages.

The Jesus of the Bible, revealing God's heart in the midst of time and culture.

Softcover: 978-0-310-27041-6

Share Your Thoughts

With the Author: Your comments will be forwarded to the author when you send them to *zauthor@zondervan.com*.

With Zondervan: Submit your review of this book by writing to *zreview@zondervan.com*.

Free Online Resources at
www.zondervan.com

Zondervan AuthorTracker: Be notified whenever your favorite authors publish new books, go on tour, or post an update about what's happening in their lives at www.zondervan.com/authortracker.

Daily Bible Verses and Devotions: Enrich your life with daily Bible verses or devotions that help you start every morning focused on God. Visit www.zondervan.com/newsletters.

Free Email Publications: Sign up for newsletters on Christian living, academic resources, church ministry, fiction, children's resources, and more. Visit www.zondervan.com/newsletters.

Zondervan Bible Search: Find and compare Bible passages in a variety of translations at www.zondervanbiblesearch.com.

Other Benefits: Register yourself to receive online benefits like coupons and special offers, or to participate in research.

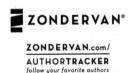